A PRACTICAL GUIDE

FOR

THE PERFUMER:

BEING A

NEW TREATISE ON PERFUMERY THE MOST FAVORABLE TO BEAUTY WITHOUT BEING INJURIOUS TO THE HEALTH,

COMPRISING A

DESCRIPTION OF THE SUBSTANCES USED IN PERFUMERY, AND THE FORMULÆ OF MORE THAN ONE THOUSAND PREPARATIONS,

SUCH AS

COSMETICS, PERFUMED OILS, TOOTH POWDERS, WATERS, EXTRACTS, TINCTURES, INFUSIONS, SPIRITS, VINEGARS, ESSENTIAL OILS, PASTILS, CREAMS, SOAPS, AND MANY NEW HYGIENIC PRODUCTS NOT HITHERTO DESCRIBED.

EDITED FROM

NOTES AND DOCUMENTS OF MESSRS. DEBAY, LUNEL, ETC.

WITH ADDITIONS

BY

PROFESSOR H. DUSSAUCE, CHEMIST,
Lately of the Laboratories of the French Government, viz., the Mining, Botanical Garden, the Imperial Manufacture of the Gobelins, the Conservatoire Impériale of Arts and Manufactures; Professor of Industrial Chemistry to the Polytechnic Institute, Paris:
Author of "A Practical Treatise on Matches, Gun-Cotton," etc., "A Complete Treatise on Tanning, Currying, and Leather Dressing," etc. etc.

PHILADELPHIA:
HENRY CAREY BAIRD,
INDUSTRIAL PUBLISHER,
406 Walnut Street.
LONDON:
TRÜBNER & CO.,
60 Paternoster Row,
1868.

PHILADELPHIA:
COLLINS, PRINTER, 705 JAYNE STREET.

PREFACE.

THE industry of the perfumer has in our day been advanced to a position which now makes it one of the first of the arts; indeed, we might almost say, one of the most useful. Perfumery has had to undergo many transformations and changes to free itself from the old beaten path of quackery and charlatanism.

In the last century, the general abuse of paints of every kind, and perfumery of different varieties, often most injurious to health, gave birth to preventives, sometimes unnecessary and exaggerated. Since, however, the perfumer, discarding a multitude of absurd receipts, now asks from the chemist combinations formed with a view to hygienic considerations, and studies the crude materials and co-ordinates them in a rational manner, perfumery has at last taken new forms in perfect harmony with good taste and refinement.

The art of the perfumer, with the advances which it has recently made, and its present scientific character, is worthy of the consideration and support of rational people. Of the truth of this assertion I hope to give a proof in this work, and unless the desire to be useful has made me the victim of a strong delusion, I trust that this guide, which has been made as complete as possible, will advantageously direct the manufacture and contribute to the progress which skilful perfumers are daily making in that interesting branch of industry.

NEW LEBANON, N. Y.,
June 19, 1868.

CONTENTS.

SECTION I.

SECTION II.

CHAPTER VI.

CHAPTER VII.

SECTION III.

CHAPTER VIII.

SECTION IV.

CHAPTER IX.

SECTION V.

CHAPTER X.

CHAPTER XI.

CHAPTER XII.

SECTION VI.

SECTION VII.

SECTION VIII.

SECTION IX.

SECTION X.

SECTION XI.

SECTION XII.

SECTION XIII.

CHAPTER XXVIII.

SECTION XIV.

CHAPTER XXIX.

CHAPTER XXX.

CHAPTER XXXI.

CHAPTER XXXII.

CHAPTER XXXIII.

SECTION XV.

CHAPTER XXXIV.

SECTION XVI.

CHAPTER XXXV.

WHITES.

CHAPTER XXXVI.

REDS.

SECTION XVII.

CHAPTER XXXVII.

CHAPTER XXXVIII.

SECTION XVIII.

CHAPTER XXXIX.

SECTION XIX.

CHAPTER XL.

CHAPTER XLI.

CHAPTER XLII.

PRACTICAL GUIDE FOR THE PERFUMER.

SECTION I.

PRELIMINARIES.

CHAPTER I.

ODORS AND PERFUMES.

An odor, in general, is an invisible, imponderable emanation, from fragrant substances. Odors cannot be propagated in the same manner as caloric and light; their movements are not submitted to the laws of reflection and refraction. They spread incessantly in the air, which is their vehicle, and follow the currents of the atmosphere.

The works of distinguished chemists and natural philosophers prove that an odor is produced by very small molecules which are disengaged from odoriferous bodies; these molecules float in the atmosphere, hanging on the different surfaces they meet, communicating to them their properties. When the odoriferous molecules are in contact with the olfactory membrane, the sense of smell is brought into action, and the brain perceives the odor. The olfactory apparatus is then indispensable to the impression of odors. For beings naturally or accidentally deprived of this organ there is no odor, just as no sounds exist for him deprived of the sense of hearing.

The odoriferous molecules or particles are of such infinitesimal tenuity that the bodies which disengage them all the time seem not to lose anything of their weight, or at least to make insensible losses; and however numerous these particles may be, an exact calculation has shown that one grain of musk had in a radius of ninety feet disengaged, in one day, 57,839,616 particles, without any diminution in its weight. This same grain of musk, abandoned to itself for six months in a large garret, communicated its odor to all the objects in the room, and being weighed in an accurate scale, it had experienced no loss.

A rose, in a few hours, can perfume 10,000 cubic feet of air, without losing in weight.

A piece of sugar on which a single drop of oil of thyme is poured, and being ground with a little alcohol, communicates the odor of thyme to 25 gallons of water.

Haller kept for forty years papers perfumed with one grain of ambergris; after this time the odor was as strong as ever. Bordenave has evaluated a molecule of camphor sensible to the smell to 2,263,584,000th of a grain. Boyle has observed that one drachm of assafœtida exposed to the open air had lost in six days the eighth part of one grain, from which Keill concludes that in one minute it had lost 1-69,120th of a grain, and, by another calculation, he demonstrates that each particle is 2·1,000,000,000,000,000th of one cubic inch. In that calculation, he supposes the particles equally distant in a sphere the radius of which is 5 feet; but as they might be more compressed towards the centre, Keill began again his calculation, and found that in that case it is necessary to multiply by 21 the number of particles, 57,839,616, given above, which produce 1,214,631,936; and he found that the volume of each particle is 38-1,000,000,000,000,000,000th.

The prodigious tenuity of odoriferous molecules made Prof. Walter think that the sensation of odors was not due to the contact of these molecules with the olfactory membrane, but to a dynamic action of the odoriferous body on the smelling sense.

Dr. Starch, of Edinburgh, has published a paper in which we find some very curious experiments on the emission and absorption of odors. According to his theory, the tissues of animal substances have more affinity for odors than vegetable tissues. The absorption of odors by outward tissues is subject to the same law that governs the absorption of caloric, that is, black tissues absorb the most odor; and this absorbing power diminishes, as the color becomes lighter, in such a manner that white tissues are those which absorb odor the least.

Odors impregnate all bodies in different degrees, and combine with nearly all the liquids. Gloves retain for a long time the perfume of ambergris; paper and cotton, that of musk. Oils and greases retain very well balsamic and volatile principles. Water, and especially alcohol, dissolve perfectly the aromatic principles of flowers. It is on this knowledge that is founded the fabrication of waters, oils, essences, pastes, pomades. Thus the perfume of flowers, so light, so fugacious, is rendered stable by art and industry. At the moment the perfume escapes from the flower, man seizes it, masters it, and uses it to increase the sum of his enjoyments.

Odoriferous bodies may be so all the time or only at certain periods. Thus some exhale their perfume in the morning, others in the middle of the day, some in the evening, and many during the night. Different circumstances may also cause the intensity of the odors to vary, such as dampness, light, heat, etc.; the addition of another substance, also, develops the strength of an odor which, alone, was nearly insensible.

The extreme subtility of odors, and the too fugacious impression they exercise on our organs, until now have been an impediment to their classification. However, some scientific men have tried to divide them into groups. Linnæus formed seven divisions:—

Aromatic,
Fragrant,
Ambrosial,
Alliaceous,
Fetid,
Repulsive,
Nauseous.

Fourcroy divides them into five groups:—

Muquous,
Fugacious oily,
Volatile oily,
Aromatic and acid,
Hydrosulphurous.

Virey, finding these classifications to be insufficient, established twenty orders, which we shall not enumerate. It has been also proposed to divide all the odors into two great classes: the *agreeable* and the *disagreeable;* but this distinction is only relative, for an odor agreeable to one person is disagreeable to another. These classifications are defective, since they make known only the quality of odors and give no idea as to their *individuality.* While chemistry has not passed any certain judgment on the existence of *primitive* odors, as has been done by natural philosophy for colors, it is, however, fair to presume that the great family of odors is reproduced by the mixture or combination of several primitive odors. It appears to us that a classification, based on the individual characteristic of odors, would be more natural. The question is, to choose, amongst odors, those which offer the most decided characteristics, and to make of them the *type*, around which analogous odors should be grouped. The different families of such a classification would bear the name of the mother odor, in such a manner that only to the family name should the odor and the different shades it produces be referred. Thus the odors which have the perfume of the rose belong to the family of the *Rosodores;* those of the musk, to the *Muskodores*, etc.

While such a classification is not perfect, it will give an idea to the reader of a classification more complete than any proposed until now:—

ROSODORES.—*Comprising all vegetables which give an odor similar to the rose.*

JASMINODORES.—*Jasmine and its substitutes.*

AURANTIODORES.—*Orange, lemon, bergamot, etc.*

MYRTODORES.—*Myrtle, pinks, etc.*

LABIODORES.—*Odors furnished by labies.*

MAGNOLIODORES.—*Badiane, anise, fennel.*

LAURINODORES.—*Camellia and succedanes.*

MENTHODORES.—*Mint and its different species.*

MUSKODORES.—*Musk, civet, castor, etc., continuing thus for all the plants, &c., with a type odor.*

We should observe that *odor* and *perfume* are

not synonymous. The former designates any agreeable or disagreeable emanation, while the latter conveys only the idea of an agreeable odor; the word perfume may at the same time designate a good odor and the substance which furnishes it; it is in this sense that incense, myrrh, ambergris, etc., are enumerated amongst perfumes.

CHAPTER II.

HISTORY OF PERFUMES.

THE use of perfumes, odors, and aromatics of every description, has been known from the most remote antiquity. The nations of Africa and Asia, Greece and Rome, were prodigal in their employ. More sensible than we to the impressions which excite to pleasure, the ancients considered sweet odors as necessary to their existence. At Athens and Corinth, the love of perfumes was so general that people assembled in perfumers' shops in the same manner as we do now in the coffee-houses. At Rome, women used such a profusion of perfumes that it was feared, for a time, that Arabia exhausted, could furnish no more, and laws were made to prevent the abuse.

In those times, the passion for perfumes was so strong that rich and poor could not do without them. They were lavished everywhere, under every circumstance; in food and drinks, in the midst of the feasts in which they celebrated Bacchus and Venus; in baths, on the body and dresses. There were no festivals, rejoicings, or funerals in which perfumes were not used. They were burned before the cradle of the newly-born infant, around the bridal bed, and on the marble of the tomb. They were offered to the gods and goddesses as a tribute and an homage; to glorify heroes, to honor kings, in temples, in the midst of palaces, in the public places, everywhere, and at all times.

Paganism which deified beauty, ugliness, virtues and vices, pleasure and love, had a very great number of gods; it comprised gods and goddesses of the first and second order, the heroes, half-gods; the numerous family of nymphs and lower divinities, the number of which exceeded *thirty-two thousand.* The prodigious number of altars arising everywhere to those divinities, the luxury of the rich and the magnificence of the feasts, the embalming of the dead, and the funerals of the rich, required an enormous quantity of perfumes.

The priests of Memphis burned, three times a day, perfumes in honor of the sun: at the rising, benzoin; at noon, myrrh; at the setting, a perfume composed of sixteen ingredients.

The disciples of Zoroaster threw six times a day perfumes on the altar on which the holy fire was kept.

At Corinth perfumes always burned around the altars of Aphrodite.

The eastern church used every year six thousand four hundred pounds of perfumes, which were collected on an area of twelve miles, and brought into Syria for the wants of the altar.

In addition to the perfumes offered to the gods, we find the aromatics employed in the preservation of the dead, and burned on funeral piles or in cassolettes during funerals.

Amongst the Egyptians, the dead were mummified, that is, preserved in such a manner that thousands of years after, the souls might resume the possession of their old bodies, which they would find in a perfect state of preservation. Such was the creed of that superstitious people; also the dead were embalmed in so perfect a manner, that corpses buried for four thousand years have been found still in a perfect state of preservation. The substances used by the Egyptians in this operation were powdered myrrh, cinnamon, aloes and some other aromatic, resinous and bituminous substances, among which we find the famous *natron*.

The Indians, Persians, Greeks, Romans, and nearly all the ancient nations of Asia and Europe, had the habit of burning their dead and collecting the ashes. It was a matter of pride for the family to cover the funeral pile with perfumes. The larger the quantity, the more honored were the dead and the family.

Around the graves of Agamemnon and Hypolyte, which exist yet, for three months perfumes and aromatics were burned.

On the occasion of the funeral of the favorite of *Alexander the Great*, the quantity of perfumes and aromatic resins burned during the transportation of the body and on the funeral pile exhausted all the stores of perfumery in India and Arabia.

Artemisia, Queen of Caria, used annually the sum of twenty thousand dollars for the purchase of the perfumes burned at the magnificent monument she had raised to the King Mausoleum, her husband.

When Sylla died, two hundred and twenty-six loads of perfumes were spread on his funeral pile.

Nero used more myrrh, cinnamon, and cassia for Poppæa's funeral than Arabia could furnish in one year.

When Pompeius entered Neapolis, cassolettes of perfumes burned in the windows of every house; and when Antony entered Alexandria to meet Cleopatra, the air was darkened by the vapors and smoke of perfumes.

The voluptuous Satraps of Asia lived all the time in an atmosphere loaded with the sweetest perfumes. The flambeaux which lighted their sumptuous parlors, in burning, spread delicious odors; their furniture was made of odoriferous woods; they mixed precious aromatics with their food and drink; artificial fountains were running in the middle of their apartments, and even on the heavy carpets they used as beds, sweet perfumes were thrown.

At a magnificent supper Otho gave to Nero, they secretly disposed in the dining-room gold and silver pipes, which poured into it aromatic vapors and costly essences. Perfumed food and drink excited the heads, and numerous smoking cassolettes completed the sweet intoxication of the senses. In this the Romans imitated the Greeks, who in all time were passionately eager for perfumes, as history teaches us. The most esteemed wines of the Athenians were those in which violets, roses, and other sweet flowers were infused. Ambreous wines, or those rendered bitter by myrrh, mastic, and aloes, were the most esteemed. But the passion for perfumes became so violent in Rome that horses, dogs, furniture, walls, etc., were rubbed with them, and their abuse was so great that a fear was entertained that there would not be enough for the use of the altar. Then, under the consulship of Licinius Crassus, a law was promulgated which restrained considerably their use, and which even specified the kind of perfume to be offered to each god or goddess.

Castus	to Saturn.
Cassia and Benzoin	to Jove.
Musk	to Juno.
Aloes	to Mars.
Saffron	to the Sun.
Mastic	to the Moon.
Cinnamon	to Mercury.
Ambergris	to Venus.

The number of substances used by the ancients as perfumes is fabulous; their mixtures, preparations, and compositions are incalculable. According to our scientific men, the Egyptians, Grecians, and Romans wrote more books on perfumes and their mixtures than the learned men of the middle ages wrote on *ontology*, which would be enormous. Some say that the immense library at Alexandria was specially composed of works on this subject.

The Greeks and Romans not only drew their perfumes from Arabia (the productions of this country would not have been sufficient), but imported aromatics and spices from India. To provide for the increasing wants of their heroes, numerous caravans started from Egypt at a certain season of the year, and went into the eastern part of Asia to fetch loads of perfumes and spices, and then came back to dispose of them in the stores of their most commercial cities—Tyre, Byblos, Smyrna, Byzance, Corinth, Alexandria, etc. The ports of these cities were always filled with merchant ships, which took these substances to transport and disperse them in the different countries of Europe.

In the following extract from an old author we find some details concerning the plants and aromatics used for funerals in antiquity:—

"When a patient had breathed his last, branches of cypress and weeping-willow were suspended to the door. The undertakers came and began to wash the corpse, then put it into a coffin trimmed with dried trunks of reed and papyrus. They covered it afterwards with perfumes composed of *incense*, *myrrh*, *anome*, *opobalsamum*, and *aloes*. The head was surrounded with a wreath of laurel, lily, white poplar, or white roses, according to the age, sex, social position, etc. It remained thus for one or two days exposed to the public. After this exposure, the corpse was placed on a funeral pile built of different resinous woods. Other perfumes, such as cassia, myrrh, incense, cinnamon, etc., were thrown into the fire to destroy the disagreeable odor disengaged by the combustion of the body. When the whole was consumed, the ashes were collected and put into an urn with different perfumes. The urn was carried in a tomb surrounded by funereal trees; and different plants, such as the violet, narcissus, and hyacinth, were sowed around and consecrated to the manes. Lastly, the friends of the dead, who accompanied the body to its last resting place, united together in a funeral feast, in which they had beans, lettuce, ache, lentils. Libations were made from cups trimmed with violets."

At the fall of the Roman Empire, this trade diminished in Europe to be concentrated in Asia. With the old civilization the law of perfumes seems to have disappeared. During the epoch when the capital of the world was invaded by barbarians, carrying with them fire and sword, luxury, the arts, and poetry took refuge in other countries, and the perfumes followed them.

However, modern civilization was throwing out its roots, and raised itself on the ruins of the old. A new era began—an era of gallantry and courtesy, in which the rights of beauty were recognized. Then women, to assure definitely their power, called perfumes to their assistance.

The taste for perfumes reappeared in the middle ages; queens and princesses spread their use around them, and to please them the lords were not long in imitating them.

At the baptism of Clovis, odoriferous candles were lighted and perfumes were burned at the doors of the church, and clouds of incense ascended in his name.

Charlemagne, after his victories, loved to rest in his palace, in which precious resins were burned. Saint Louis loved perfumes, and used to say in the plains of Palestine, "Oh, delicious country of Arabia! I long for thy conquest, to offer to the Lord thy myrrh and incense!"

In the pomps of the Catholic Church, which, in its processions, were so magnificently developed, perfumes and flowers occupied the first rank.

Amongst the high lords of the middle ages, the hands and mouth were washed after meals with rose water; the rich had fountains pouring out aromatic waters to perfume their dining-rooms.

At a feast given by *Philip the Good*, Duke of

Burgundy, opposite the table was the statue of a child which was throwing off rose water.

Under Louis XV. the ladies who frequented the court adopted every day a new perfume, in such manner that the rooms in the palace were one day perfumed with tuberose, next day with amber or aloes, and the following days by other perfumes. The variety of these sweet odors, the art of spreading them on the clothes, so as not to offend the sense of smell, gave to that court the name of *the perfumed court.*

Since that time perfumes have become a necessity to the toilet. The art of perfumery, to which chemistry has given so much help, knows how to fix the most fugitive odors, and offer them under a multitude of forms, the sweetness of which testifies to the salubrity of their use.

CHAPTER III.

MANIPULATIONS. DECOCTION—INFUSION—DISSOLUTION—MACERATION —FILTRATION — DECANTATION—DISCOLORATION — EPURATION—DISTILLATION—CONSERVATION AND DRYING OF FLOWERS—BLEACHING OF SPONGES—CONSERVATION OF PERFUMES.

Decoction.

An operation which consists in boiling in a liquid an organic substance, so as to extract its active principles. Water saturated with the active principles of the substance, is called a *decoction.* The decoction is different from the infusion. In the infusion the water is poured while boiling on the organic substances to be exhausted, while in the decoction the substance is boiled with the water. Each operation gives a different result, a plant does not yield the same principles by decoction as by infusion. By decoction, the extractive, resinous, and bitter principles are obtained, while by infusion a larger quantity of aromatic and volatile principles, essences, etc., are extracted. These principles may produce on the animal economy an effect which differs from that which results from those obtained by decoction. It is then very important not to confound them.

The time of the ebullition is regulated by the nature of the substance treated by decoction. Leaves, and especially flowers, ought to be exposed only to a short ebullition if they are odoriferous; roots and aromatic barks should be subjected to a short ebullition, because the aromatic principles evaporate and are decomposed by the action of heat, or are dissipated. Consequently, it is very important in the preparation of decoctions, to know the way boiling water acts on the different substances, so as to discontinue the operation at the proper time.

Infusion.

Infusion consists in pouring a boiling liquid on an organic substance, so as to extract the principles, and when cool, to separate the product by decantation or filtration. (See *Decoction.*)

Dissolution.

The operation by which a liquid body communicates that state to any other body, whatever is its nature. The dissolution is also called *solution.* Any body which disappears in water or some other liquid, without destroying its transparency, is soluble, and the liquid which contains it is called a dissolution. In this state the body has not lost its primitive properties. Sugar, dissolved in water, has the same sweet taste which characterized it when solid. Water is a precious solvent in the sense that bodies dissolved in it retain their properties. Insoluble bodies render liquids muddy, being deposited after a time more or less long, and form what is called a *precipitate* or *deposit.* However, we must not consider as insoluble all the bodies which render water muddy. Very few substances are absolutely insoluble, for the most insoluble, such as sulphate of baryta, chloride of silver, &c., are sensibly soluble; truly, the quantity of water is so great that under ordinary circumstances they may be considered as insoluble. Amongst soluble substances we must not rank those which decompose in water and form new products which are soluble. The dissolution, in separating the molecules, divides bodies so as to weaken those properties which would be too energetic in the solid state. The dissolution offers the best example of the great divisibility of matter. Gases dissolve in proportion to the pressure they are subjected to, while solid substances are generally more soluble in warm than cold water. Lime, magnesia, and zircona are exceptions to the rule. A liquid which has dissolved a substance in so great a quantity that it cannot dissolve any more of the same substance under ordinary circumstances, is called a *saturated solution.* When a substance is more soluble in a warm than in cold liquid, the dissolution saturated at the ordinary temperature will dissolve a larger quantity when warm, then it is *super saturated,* and when allowed to stand and cool slowly, the excess of the soluble body is deposited, and the molecules assume peculiar geometrical forms called *crystals.*

Maceration.

An operation which consists in allowing to stay together for some time, at the ordinary temperature, a solid substance and a liquid, for the purpose of dissolving some of its immediate principles, or to extract the soluble principles, or, lastly, to preserve them.

Filtration.

An operation which consists in passing a liquid through a porous body, which retains the solid substances. It has for its object to clarify the liquid, or to collect the solid bodies mixed with it, or to attain these two results at the same time. Sometimes the filter is a piece of felt, or a frame covered with a piece of woollen or cotton cloth, or even a piece of filtering paper; sometimes it is composed of vessels with several bottoms, pierced with holes and covered with one or several beds of straw, cotton, sand, or charcoal. Generally, it is necessary that the filtering substance should be porous, or so divided as to let the liquid pass and retain the foreign bodies which are suspended in it.

Decantation.

An operation, the object of which is to separate a liquid from solid substances deposited in it. To decant, pour slowly, sloping little by little, the vessel containing the liquid; but in our judgment it is better to use a siphon.

Discoloration

Has for its object to remove the color from vegetable and animal substances. Generally, liquids are discolorized by two processess: by *animal charcoal* or by *chlorine*. *Animal charcoal* comprises two varieties: The *animal black*, or bone black, prepared from bones of different animals; and *ivory black*, prepared by the calcination of small pieces of ivory. This black, which is very light, bright, lamellose, friable, and difficult to incinerate, has the property of discolorizing many liquid and solid substances. It is used principally in refining sugar.

To use it in the laboratory it has to be purified by washings with distilled water; sometimes it is treated with one-fifth of its weight of hydrochloric acid and washing afterwards with boiling distilled water.

Chlorine in a gaseous or liquid state, on account of its affinity for hydrogen, destroys vegetable and animal coloring matters. It also destroys odoriferous substances, miasms, etc. Fumigations of chlorine gas irritate the respiratory organs, and, if practised in closed places, may produce unpleasant consequences. Chlorine has been substituted by aspersions of *chlorides*, which are mixtures of *chlorides* and *hypochlorites.*

Epuration.

This word indicates two operations—1st. *Purification* or *Clarification*, which is effected spontaneously when the aqueous, acid, or oily juices expressed from vegetables are allowed to stand until they deposit their impurities, or until by a slight fermentation they throw off these impurities by floating them to the surface. 2d. *Refining.* In perfumery, the greases which constitute the bases for pomades are refined, that is, made very white by adding to them seven or eight grains of tartaric acid per pound, and then beating them with a small broom.

Distillation.

The operation by which liquids are converted into vapor by the help of heat, and this vapor is condensed by cooling. The principal object of this operation is to separate liquids from fixed substances, or from those having a different degree of volatility. The distillation is effected in a peculiar apparatus called an *alembic.* The cucurbit, the head, and the refrigeratory, constitute the three essential parts of the alembic, and by their form exercise a notable influence on the results of the operation. The *cucurbit*, or lower part, in which are placed the substances to be distilled, ought to be constructed in such a manner as to present to the action of heat the largest surface possible. The bottom is convex, which disposition is more advantageous than flat or concave bottoms. It must be very wide. The *head*, the object of which is to conduct the vapors from the cucurbit to the refrigeratory, has been the object of many changes since its origin. At first it received too considerable a development, and was then exposed to be too rapidly cooled; the result was that the vapors were condensed in it and fell back into the cucurbit, thus rendering the operation much slower. To remedy this imperfection, the neck of the head was made with a kind of gutter, which received the condensed vapors and brought them to the running pipe. It has been found necessary to make the head very small. It is simply formed of a covered copper pipe, of which one end is exactly adapted to the opening of the cucurbit, while the smaller is adjusted to the refrigeratory. However, a head thus disposed must not be too small, and the lower opening especially ought to be large enough to present little resistance to the vapors which rise into it. The *refrigeratory* is the part in which the vapors condense and resume the liquid form. In the old alembics it simply consisted of a straight pipe, passing through a wooden box full of water or ice. But the space was not large enough, and the condensation was imperfect, and this pipe was then substituted by a worm or spiral pipe, surrounded by cold water.

Distillation is one of the most important branches of the perfumer's art, since it has for its object the production of essential oils, essences, odoriferous waters, vinegars, &c. Thus, on account of the volatility and delicacy of the substances, the alembic is the principal and the most useful instrument of the laboratory of the perfumer.

Conservation and Drying of Flowers.

Plants must be collected in clear and dry weather, after sunrise, at the moment the flower begins to blossom; they are to be separated from earth, grass, leaves, etc.

Some are dried in the shade on cloth or on frames suspended from a wall, some are dried in the oven, and others in a baker's oven, etc. All these processes are defective.

Recently it has been tried to keep plants by Mason's process, that is, by a progressive desiccation under strong pressure, but this operation destroys the appearance of the plant and renders adulteration more easy. The best method is that used by M. Violand, of Colmar (France). The building he employs is 180 feet long; it has three stories. The drying rooms are established in the second and third stories; the first is the store-room. In the store-room are on each side large boxes hermetically closed, and containing each 1000 pounds of the dried plants. In the second story are three ranks of wooden lattice-work, separated in all the length by passages which permit free access to the frames. Superposed, one on the other, are ten frames for the second story, and fifteen for the third, at a distance of 1½ foot from each other. This space is more than sufficient for the renewing of the air, and to permit the men to put up or take off the plants. Spread on the frames, 6 feet long and 3 feet wide, the plants dry admirably and quickly. Their surfaces being entirely exposed to the air, there is no necessity for turning them over, as in the old process, which required from 3 to 4 weeks, but is now done in from 36 to 48 hours. By this method the leaves keep their forms and do not fall into powder in drying.

The walls of the drying-room are made of wood; they are pierced at regular intervals with openings, destined to renew the air. These openings are closed or opened at will so as to regulate the drying-room when the air is too damp.

The dispositions are the same for the upper story, only the number of frames is greater.

These drying-rooms are among the most useful and ingenious conceptions of our times, and it would be a great improvement if all perfume manufacturers adopted them.

Bleaching of Sponges.

Sponge is a production of the sea, about the nature of which naturalists have not always agreed. Some look on it as belonging to the animal kingdom; others classify it amongst vegetables, and some make of it a kind of polypary made by zoophytes.

Sponge presents itself in the form of a mass of fibrous tissues more or less dense, flexible, and elastic, capable of absorbing water, and coated while living with a half-fluid gelatinous substance.

Sponge exhausted by ether, alcohol, and hydrochloric acid contains

Carbon	47.16
Hydrogen	6.31
Oxygen	26.90
Nitrogen	16.15
Iodine	1.07
Sulphur	0.09
Phosphorus	1.90

Before being employed for the uses of the toilet, or even for certain domestic uses, sponges as extracted from the sea require the following preparations:—

1. Dipping them for six or seven days in cold

water, being careful to change the water several times daily, and each time press the sponge in the hands.

2. Disembarrass them of the small stones they contain by macerating them for 24 hours in the following mixture:—

Hydrochloric acid . .	1 part.
Water	20 parts.

3. Wash them several times in pure water, and dip them in sulphuric acid.

4. Repeat this immersion for four days, being careful to press them from time to time.

5. Leave them 24 hours in running water, and dry them in the air and the shade.

Conservation of Perfumes.

Perfumes must be kept in closed vessels to assure a good state of conservation. Objects to be exported to warm countries should be of the first quality, so as to resist atmospheric variations. It is a known fact that the sea air, excessive heat, and thunder storms decompose perfumes of the second quality.

Pomades should not be exposed to the sun, which melts them, nor to dampness, which renders them musty.

Perfumed waters containing alcohol are easily kept, and even become better by growing old.

Toilet soaps, rose powders, tooth powders, vegetable red (rouge), white of pearl, ought to be kept in a dry place.

Toilet and other vinegars, rose milks, and virginal creams, ought to be protected from the frost.

Distilled waters should be kept in a cool place protected from the contact of the air and light. The bottles must be entirely filled and well closed with glass stoppers. Some very aromatic waters, such as those of orange flower, roses, peppermint, preserve their aroma for a long time by only covering with paper or parchment the opening of the vessels which contain them. Others, as anis, fennel, etc., lose their odor in a short time when kept in open bottles.

Waters distilled from odorless plants are rapidly decomposed by contact with the air. A very important fact to be observed is that distilled waters must be kept in bottles which have been previously washed with pure water, the smallest quantity of river or fountain water occasions sometimes in compound distilled waters a kind of alteration which develops in them a gelatinous substance not yet examined, but similar to pectic acid in consistency.

CHAPTER IV.

ENUMERATION AND DESCRIPTION OF THE MOST USUAL PERFUMES.

THE sweetest flowers, the perfumes, and generally all aromatic substances are produced in Eastern countries. However, some are collected in temperate climates, which have a fugitive and sweet odor. The three kingdoms of nature furnish odors, but the vegetable kingdom excels the two others in number, variety, and sweetness.

From all the substances used in perfumery, we shall name only the perfumes and aromatics most in use.

OF ANIMAL ORIGIN.	OF VEGETABLE ORIGIN.		
Musk,	Amber,	Gelanga Root,	
Civet,	Incense,	Leaves,	Of different small and large vegetables. (Leaves, Flowers, Fruits, Seeds)
Castoreum,	Myrrh,	Flowers,	
Ambergris.	Benzoin,	Fruits,	
	Storax,	Seeds,	
	Mastic,	Nutmegs,	
	Bdellium,	Vanilla,	
	Labdanum,	Cloves,	
	Liquidambar,	Ginger,	
	Balsams of Tolu,	Anise,	
	" Mecca,	Ambrette,	
	Rose-wood,	Thyme,	

OF ANIMAL ORIGIN.	OF VEGETABLE ORIGIN.	
	Sandal wood,	Origanum,
	Aloes "	Lavander,
	Cedar "	Cardamom,
	Sassafras "	Angelica,
	Ceylon Cinnamon,	Rose,
	Cassia,	Heliotrope,
	Lemon Peel,	Jasmine,
	Orange Peel,	Lily,
	Bergamot,	Tuberose,
	Suchet Root,	Rue,
	Calamus Aromaticus, etc. etc.	

Musk.

An animal secretion of a brown color found in excretory follicles about the navel of a male ruminant, called *musk-deer*, found in China, Tonquin, Thibet, and Tartary. Musk is one of the strongest odoriferous substances; it is very lasting; its odor adheres to all the substances around it. In spasmodic affections, when musk is given internally, it exhales through the pores of the skin and impregnates the transpiration with a musky odor. It is said that the effect of the odor of musk on living animals is so violent that hunters will bleed at the nose, if they neglect certain precautions when depriving the animal of his bag.

The musk has the singular property of being deprived of its odor when mixed with milk of lime, cherry-laurel water, ergot, mustard oil, etc. Mineral kermes gives it the odor of onions. New experiments will probably bring to light a great many other combinations.

According to the analyses of MM. Guibourt and Blondeau, musk contains: *water*, *ammonia*, *stearin*, *elain*, *cholesterin*, *an acid combined with ammonia*, *peculiar volatile oil*, *hydrochlorate of lime*, *carbonate of lime*, *gelatine*, *fibrin*, *phosphate of lime*, *hairs*, *sand*, *salt of lime*, *organic acid*, *etc.*

Chemistry has already succeeded in preparing a kind of artificial musk. In Germany they have manufactured it for some time, by treating one part of essential oil of amber by four parts of nitric acid. A kind of yellow rosin, having the odor of musk, is obtained. The odor of musk is met with also in man and several animals. Alexander the Great, and the learned Haller, transpired the odor of musk. The buffalo, several kinds of rats, deer, antelope, and many other animals, emit the smell of musk during the season of rutting. Amongst birds, ducks, owls, and pelicans. Amongst the reptiles, some snakes, crocodiles, and some species of turtles; and many insects exhibit the same phenomenon. A multitude of plants possess the odor of musk in different degrees. Lastly, the excrements of some animals, such as the skunk, coon, etc., have a musky odor.

Musk is rarely ever used alone. Its penetrating and tenacious odor may affect the nerves, causing some persons to faint, and sometimes occasions convulsions; but this perfume being mixed in very small quantities with some others, such as the ambergris, lavander, etc., loses its offensive smell and becomes agreeable to the olfactories.

The trade distinguishes three kinds of musk. The *China musk* or *Tonquin;* the *Bengal musk*, which comprises the *Thibet;* and the *Tartary musk.*

The China musk is divided into three classes; the first, called *musk of the royal hunt*, is in flat bladders, sometimes ovoids, round; sometimes long, dried, thin, soft to the touch, of a weight varying from one drachm to one ounce. The upper part of each bladder, which is pierced in the middle by a little hole, is covered with long hairs, of a reddish color, thicker on the edges than on the middle, and around the entire circumference; the lower part has no hairs; it bears on the middle a red mark. Its appearance is whitish-gray. The color of the musk contained in this envelop is dark brown. It is viscous to the touch; its odor is penetrating and subtle; if weakened, it ought not to be ammoniacal nor empyreumatic. This kind is very rare in commerce. This musk is exported in lead or tin boxes weighing from sixteen to twenty-one ounces. Each bladder is enveloped in China paper (tissue-paper), which bears a seal and the name of the place it comes from. To this first envelope succeeds another formed of Chinese varnished paper, and covered with a coating of tar.

The second kind has about the same properties

as the first; its odor is less pure; it is a little ammoniacal. It is exported, 1, in entire bladders, often bearing a seal similar to the above; 2, in bladders which have been opened, and do not bear a seal. The packings used are the same. The third kind is contained in bladders of various shapes. The hair which covers them is less abundant on the edges; they are damp, thicker than the others, and are always sewed. The product they contain is heavier, it crushes and dries more easily; its odor is fetid and ammoniacal, and the true odor of musk is developed only after some time. Its perfume is less delicate. This musk is exported in lead or tin boxes, weighing from four to six pounds. The Bengal musk is nearly similar to the Tonquin, but its odor is not so delicate, and is somewhat ammoniacal. The bladders which contain it, generally, are not so well closed, often sewed over, damp. The hair which covers the skin is not so long, and is mixed. The bladders have not at their upper part the small hole we remark on the Tonquin; the skin also is thicker. It is exported in lead or tin boxes weighing from twenty ounces to six pounds.

The musk of Tartary is in flat, dry, and long bladders. The skin is thick, the upper part is covered with short hairs of a whitish-gray color; the appearance of the lower part is a dirty gray. The musk it contains is compact, and has a fibrous consistency. Its odor is little penetrating, ammoniacal, and easily evaporates.

Falsification.—A substance as costly as musk cannot be brought from its place of production without being adulterated. Thus a great many things have been tried to sophisticate the precious product; dried blood has been mixed with it, various animal substances, resins, wax, pieces of skin, hairs, iron, sand, and many other things. A microscopical examination will detect the metallic and earthy parts; the incineration also leaves these substances. By passing a red hot iron through adulterated musk, the odor of resins, wax, and other animal or vegetable substances can be detected. For all the trials a specimen type should be examined at the same time. Good musk is very soluble in water, does not present hard substances when pressed between the fingers; it colors paper reddish-brown.

Civet.

The name civet is given to all unctuous products extracted from a cavity, more or less deep, placed below the anus of the civet (*viverra civetta*), and opening by the outside. That cavity, in the bottom of which we meet two glandular receptacles, contains a fatty matter similar to musk, of a buttery consistence; at first of a whitish color, which becomes brown by time; of a strong odor, which is sometimes fetid; of a burning and acrid taste. This substance, also called civet, is much used in perfumery. Civets are found in Asia and Africa, principally in Abyssinia, Guinea, and Congo. The civet is extracted from the body of the living animal by carefully introducing a little spoon into the receptacle which contains it. The Amsterdam civet is preferred to that of the East or India; that from Guinea would be the best if it was not adulterated with storax, or some other odoriferous substance. The civet received from Asia is extracted from the *Zibet*, an animal having great analogy with the civet, but different in some peculiar characteristics. Lavender, thyme, and other scented waters acquire much superiority when prepared with a small quantity of civet.

Civet enters into the fabrication of several compound perfumes, among them the powder of Chypre; it is used also by tobacconists to perfume snuff. Civet is adulterated with honey, lard, rancid butter, and other fatty bodies—blood, sand, earth; then the product has not its genuine color, odor, or consistency, and contains often grains more or less hard—characteristics not possessed by a specimen of genuine civet.

Castoreum.

An animal substance with a very strong odor, often secreted in a pocket that the beaver (*castor fiber*) carries under the tail. Castoreum is now very little used in perfumery, but in medicine it is employed successfully as a powerful anti-spasmodic.

Amber (Succinum).

(Arabic, *ambar*), "A fossil, indurated, vegetable juice, transparent or translucent, sometimes colorless, but usually of some shade of yellow or brown, and negatively electrified by friction." *Eng. Cyclop.*

Amber.

A mineral substance, hard, brittle, susceptible of a fine polish, and a color more or less yellow; more highly esteemed when whitish; its specific gravity varies from 1.080 to 1.085. Its taste is not agreeable, has no odor, but acquires some by rubbing it. Amber, exposed to the fire, becomes soft, melts and burns, giving out at the same time an agreeable odor.

Amber is generally associated with deposits of combustibles in earths of recent formation. It is met in arenaceous matters which accompany *lignites*, and often in contact with it. When associated with fossil woods, it is generally adhering to the vertical parts. This observation would prove that amber is nothing else than a transformation of a resinous substance produced by those vegetables which now belong to the mineral kingdom. Amber is found in France. Three or four millions of pounds are generally imported from the coasts of the Baltic Sea, where are found the most celebrated deposits. From Dantzig to Memel the export of amber is the object of a considerable industry. It is found in beds of sand, stone, and fossil woods. Generally it is in little nodules; however, sometimes considerable masses are met with. Recently there was discovered, between Memel and Konigsberg, a specimen weighing twenty-five pounds. It is insoluble in water, soluble in alcohol, or in a solution of subcarbonate of potash; melted in siccative linseed oil, and incorporated with spirits of turpentine, it furnishes a very good varnish.

Ambergris (Ambra grisea).

The origin of this substance was for a long time unknown. It is considered now to be a secretion formed in the intestines of some cachalots, principally the *Physeter macrocephalus.* It is found in irregular masses, and sometimes in large quantities, floating on the waters of the sea, or thrown on the shore of the coasts of Coromandel, Sumatra, in China, Japan, on the coasts of Africa and Brazil, Madagascar, Sicily, etc. It is formed in concentric layers. Its fracture is shelly, covered with gray spots, mixed with black, yellow, and white points. It is opalescent, of a variable consistency, sometimes soft and tenacious, sometimes hard and brittle, returning, however, the impression of the nail. Its taste is greasy. Its odor is strong but agreeable, and it is principally disengaged by heat and rubbing.

Ambergris has been sometimes found in very large pieces. The Dutch Company bought one piece from the King of Tidor which weighed one hundred and seventy-four pounds. He sold it for three thousand four hundred dollars. This same piece was sold in Europe for twenty-two thousand dollars. The French Company in India bought a ball weighing two hundred and thirty-seven and a half pounds for ten thousand four hundred dollars. This substance was so common years ago in the islands of the Polynesia that the inhabitants of Timor used it to calk their canoes.

Several chemists have found ambergris to consist of—

Ambreine	52.7
Resin	30.8
Benzoic acid	1.1
Carbonaceous substance	5.4

Ambergris softens by heat, and when melted constitutes a thick oil, blackish, very volatile. It burns with rapidity, and gives a bright flame. It is insoluble in water, very soluble in alcohol, ethers, and some fixed oils.

Ambergris is rarely used alone. It is by mixing it with some other perfumes that its odor is developed. The *essence of amber* of perfumers is an alcoholic tincture of ambergris, to which oils of roses, cloves, lavender, &c. are added. The perfume known by the name of *essence of civet* is obtained by the maceration, in a quart of rectified alcohol, of—

Civet	4 drachms.
Ambergris . . .	2 "

After three days of maceration it is filtered, and kept in well-corked bottles.

It is by pouring a few drops of this tincture into scented waters, tooth-powders, soaps, &c., that an ambrosial odor is given them.

The greatest consumption of ambergris is in compounding waters and perfumes for the toilet; nevertheless, medicine uses it sometimes in the atony of some of the organs.

Ambrette

Is also called *musk seed*, and belongs to a species of *Ketmie*, a plant belonging to the family of the *Malvaces.* It is the odoriferous ketmie (*Hibiscus-el-moschus*), which is found in the East Indies, and in the warm countries of America, that furnishes the ambrette. The pod which contains it is pyramidal, about two inches long. The flowers are yellow, with a purple bottom; the calyx falls before the flower.

Ambrette is used in perfumery on account of its odor, which partakes at the same time of that of musk and vanilla. It was the perfume generally used for hair powder.

That seed is found to contain:—

Water and ligneous matter .	52.00
Mucilage	36.00
Albuminous matter . . .	5.60
Fixed oils, Concrete matter, Odoriferous substance, Colored resin,	6.40
	100.00

Resin.

A proximate principle of vegetables, composed of *oxygen*, *hydrogen*, and *carbon*. Resins are solid, brittle, odorless, insipid, or acrid substances; a little heavier than water, yellowish, and more or less transparent. All can be electrified negatively by rubbing; they are bad conductors of electricity. At the ordinary temperature the air is without action on them. They are insoluble in water, soluble in alcohol, ether, fixed and volatile oils. There exist remarkable differences in the resins, according to their origin. They may be divided into three classes, viz: the liquid, solid, and gummy resins. They are also distinguished as natural and artificial. Many of them exude from the trunks and branches of trees.

Liquid resins are excretive products of vegetables of an inflammable nature, having a consistency between volatile oils and dry resins; the best known are the balsams of Canada, copaiba, Mecca, pitch, the liquid resin of larch, the turpentines of Chio, Venice, etc.

Solid resins are pitch, resin, white pitch, liquid storax, sandarac, benzoin, dragon's blood, etc.

Gummy resins are the Ammoniac bdellium, galbanum, assafœtida, elemi, labdanum, etc.

Resins are much used, either in the arts or in perfumery. We shall describe the most important.

Benzoin.

A resinous and inflammable substance, with a very pleasant odor, obtained by making incisions in the trunk of *Styrax benzoin.* It is imported from the Philippine Islands and Sumatra. Two kinds are known in commerce: one, which is the purest, is called *amygdaloid benzoin,* because it is formed of whitish drops, half transparent, oval, similar to almonds, coated by a reddish concrete juice, granular, and very brittle. The other species is the *common benzoin,* of a darker color, more opalescent, coarser in its texture, and does not present the drops observed in the above. It is the one most usually employed in perfumery and the arts.

Amygdaloid benzoin is in compact masses, formed of a multitude of agglomerated drops; its fracture is white, when recent, yellow or reddish when more or less old. It is on account of its form that it is designated by the name of *amygdaloid.* Sometimes it is also met with in separated drops, flat, and long, yellowish outside, white inside, and having the appearance of an almond.

Amygdaloid benzoin has the odor of vanilla; that imported from Siam is the sweetest. Perfumers dissolve it in alcohol, and prepare a tincture which enters into the composition of many preparations. The cosmetic known by the name of *virginal milk* is a simple tincture of benzoin.

Common benzoin is a reunion of drops mixed with ligneous and earthy substances, which give to the mass, when broken, a light-grayish appearance, spotted with white. Another kind is also met with, the fracture of which is reddish.

The characteristics which distinguish benzoin from other resinous substances, and which place it in the first class of natural resinous balsams, are, that it contains a peculiar acid, to which the name of *benzoic* has been given; united to resinous matter, and is more odoriferous than the resins properly so called. It is also partly soluble in water, and completely so in alcohol.

According to Bucholz, benzoin is found to be composed of *resin*, *benzoic acid*, *a substance similar to Peruvian balsam*, *an aromatic principle soluble in water and alcohol*, and *ligneous detritus.*

It has been thought for a long time that benzoic acid existed only in the resin of that name. Now this acid is easily extracted from some other substances, in which its presence was hitherto unknown. Thus the balsams of Tolu, Peru, and others; castoreum, vanilla, elm-bark, the oil of bitter-almonds, etc., give a benzoic acid similar to that extracted from benzoin.

The most simple manner of obtaining the *flowers of benzoin*, or benzoic acid, is the following: Spread, uniformly, powdered benzoin in a cast-iron kettle; a cone is made of very smooth pasteboard, which is applied and pasted on the edges of the kettle. At the top of the cone is an opening, closed with tissue paper. The apparatus being thus arranged, the kettle is heated over a sand-bath, and the heat is kept up for a few hours. The benzoic acid is volatilized, and adheres to the edges of the cone in the form of white needles, while the steam escapes through the tissue paper.

A benzoin is found in the trade which is deprived of its benzoic acid by an ebullition in ordinary water, or in lime-water. This fraud is detected by the feebleness of the odor, and the sweet, balsamic taste of the product.

Myrrh.

A gum resin imported from Arabia and Abyssinia, furnished, it is thought, by the *Laurus myrrhæ.* Myrrh is solid, reddish; its fracture is bright, and very friable. It is found in the trade in smooth pieces, but much oftener rough. It is principally when reduced to powder, and mixed with some other substances, that myrrh exhales a most agreeable odor.

This gum resin is tonic, antiperiodic, and balsamic; it enters into several pharmaceutical preparations. Sacred history teaches us that Eastern nations looked on myrrh as one of the most precious productions of the earth. In Moses' time and before, it was burned on altars, mixed with benzoin. Myrrh was one of the presents brought by the three kings to Christ at the time of his birth.

Labdanum.

A resin which naturally exudes from the *Cretan cystei.* Purified from all heterogeneous substances this resin has a thick consistency; its color is brown or blackish; its odor, when developed, is analogous to that of the ambergris. It is not much used in perfumery now, but its use in soaps and fatty bodies would give excellent results.

Mastic.

An aromatic resin, of a white and transparent color, furnished by the tree called lentisk. Eastern nations used this resin as a cosmetic; women chose it to whiten their teeth and perfume the breath.

Incense.

An aromatic gum resin, which, in burning, gives out a perfumed vapor. The incense received from Africa and Arabia exudes from a kind of juniper-tree peculiar to those countries. That from India exudes from the tree called *Boswellia;* it is in yellow tears, round, and larger than the grains of the African incense. The African incense is in reddish tears, and in irregular pieces more or less reddish. The first are round, with a tarnished and waxy fracture. They become soft under the teeth; they have an aromatic taste, which is a little acrid. Incense in lumps has a stronger taste and odor than that in tears. It is often mixed with detritus of bark, and contains small crystals of carbonate of lime. The Indian incense is nearly entirely formed of round, yellow, half-tarnished tears; this is of a remarkable purity; it is abundantly found in commerce.

Incense is partially soluble in alcohol and water; it melts with difficulty by heat, burns with a fine white flame, and gives a whitish, abundant, and fuliginous flame, the odor of which is agreeable and penetrating.

The analysis of incense gives—

Resin	56
Yellow, volatile oil, with the odor of lemon	5
Gum	30
Carbonate and sulphate of potash, chloride of potassium, phosphate and carbonate of lime	9
	100

Balsams.

Balsams are aromatic substances, of one-half liquid consistency, which naturally exude from different trees. They differ from resins in their consistency. Resins are dry and friable, while balsams belong to the class of the soft and oleaginous substances, and possess all the balsamic properties. Chemical analysis has found that *benzoic* and *cinnamic acids*, *resin* and *volatile oil*, enter into their composition.

It is in Arabia, and amongst Eastern nations that balsams and balsamic compounds were originally used. During the Crusades, balsams began to be introduced into Europe. Generally they were believed to be very efficacious for the cure of wounds. Now, perfumers find in balsams the basis of many cosmetics, either liquid or solid. The greater part of those balsams which are burned in cassolettes are nothing but a mixture of balsams with some resinous or aromatic substances, such as benzoin, vanilla, &c. The most employed in perfumery are—

CANADA BALSAM, or *white balsam*. It is very transparent, has the same fluidity as turpentine, from which it differs only in its odor, which is sweeter, and analogous to that of lemon or Mecca balsam. It is extracted in Canada from a kind of fur tree called *Balsam of Gilead*, MECCA BALSAM (or *Judea*). It is a resin which exudes from a tree growing in Arabia the Happy. The true Mecca balsam, which is very rare, is limpid and whitish, acrid, aromatic, and very penetrating.

BALSAM OF PERU.—A balsamic resin, obtained by the decoction of branches and leaves of the *Myroxylon peruiferum*, which grows in the warmest parts of South America, principally in Peru. It is transparent, of a consistency similar to that of boiled syrup. Its color is of a very dark reddish-brown; its odor agreeable and penetrating.

BALSAM OF TOLU.—A balsamic resin known in commerce by the name of American balsam, produced by a species of *Myroxylon*, which grows principally in the province of Carthagena, in the neighborhood of the town of Tolu. This balsam has a soft consistency, a gilded, greenish-yellow color; an agreeable aromatic taste, a sweet smell, analogous to that of benzoin.

Storax.

A resinous gum obtained from the incision of the *Storax officinale*, a tree growing in Caramania, Syria, and some other localities of Asia Minor. There are two kinds, one solid and the other liquid. The perfection of storax depends on its whiteness. As soon as liquid storax is collected, the edges of the incision made in the tree are scraped, and from this operation results another kind of storax of inferior quality. They are mixed. The storax thus mixed is brought from

Caramania and the island of Cyprus. It is introduced into large kettles, and by means of fire and stirring, it is separated from the earthy parts and other impurities. Thus cleansed, it is put into bags, and exported in that condition. The dry or solid storax is a resinous substance, of which there are two kinds in commerce—the calamite storax, and the common storax.

The calamite is in masses formed of amygdaloid drops, of a yellowish-white color, soft, opalescent, voluminous, reunited by a brown reddish substance, forming a vitreous and transparent coating. Its odor is sweet. Its taste is aromatic, perfumed, and a little acrid. It is dry and friable. The second kind, or the common storax, has a soft consistency, a reddish color, fat. It is in irregular masses, dry, brittle, light, full of small bright particles; it has an agreeable odor, but less penetrating than the above.

Camphor.

Camphor is now considered by chemists as one of the immediate principles of a great many vegetables, among which we name ginger, cinnamon, sassafras, zedoary, galanga, cardamom, and others of the same family; it is met with also in the Labies, such as lavander, thyme, rosemary, hyssop, etc.

There are several varieties of camphor, but the two most common in commerce are those of Japan and China; the latter is the most esteemed. The tree which produces camphor is the *Laurus camphora* or camphor tree. The process for obtaining it is very simple. The branches of the tree are cut in small pieces, boiled in water, and as the ebullition progresses, the camphor floats on the surface. When the water has removed all the camphor, it is passed through a sieve, allowed to cool, and thus the solidified camphor is collected. Thus obtained, it is in a crude state, and must be purified; for this purpose it is mixed with a little lime, and sublimed in vessels with flat bottoms over a sand-bath.

Refined camphor is moulded in cakes weighing from two to four pounds. It is very white; unctuous to the touch; its fracture is bright; it has a peculiar penetrating odor; it can be powdered only when mixed with a little alcohol or ether. It is soluble in alcohol, ethers, fixed and volatile oils, greases, melted resin, etc.

An artificial camphor is manufactured by passing a slow current of hydrochloric acid gas through spirit of turpentine, kept at a low temperature. The gas is absorbed, and, after a certain time, a white substance, having the odor of camphor, is deposited. This substance is the *chlorhydrate of camphene*, or *artificial camphor*.

Camphor is used in perfumery to flavor soaps, tooth powders, sachets, and other preparations.

Wood and Resin of Aloes.

This very odoriferous wood is imported from China and the island of Socotora. It is found in the market in small pieces of five or six inches. It is sufficient to rub it to have it give an agreeable odor; when burned, it gives an aromatic smoke.

In ancient times aloes was used in religious ceremonies and for the preservation of dead bodies. It was the basis of the famous panacea of Paracelsus, who pretended to have discovered the secret of prolonging human life beyond its natural limits.

Aloes-wood in China takes the place of the compound perfumes we burn in houses under the name of odoriferous candles.

Sandal-wood

Is the name given in the trade to three kinds of woods imported from the East Indies. We distinguish the *yellowish sandal*, the *white sandal*, and the *red sandal.*

The *yellowish sandal* is heavy and compact, with straight fibres; its color is yellowish, its taste bitter, its odor is as a mixture of musk, lemon, and rose. A volatile oil, with a very strong odor, is extracted from this wood by distillation. The *white sandal* differs from the above only by its color and its odor, which is weaker. The *red sandal* is dense and heavy; its fibres are sometimes straight, sometimes undulated. It has no sensible odor. Its taste is slightly astringent. The *yellowish sandal* is the only one used in perfumery. In the East it is burned in cassolettes. The Chinese mix it with rice-paste to make perfumed candles. In Europe it is used only to make perfumery boxes, etc.

Rosewood.

This wood is thus called on account of its color and odor. It is furnished by several trees in different countries—in the Canaries, the Antilles, Jamaica, Cayenne, and also in China. This wood has the odor and color of the rose. It is without sap-wood, covered with a thin coating, compact, a fine grain, of a pale or yellowish color, with veins of a bright or blackish red. Generally it is more or less hollow. It is used in perfumery.

Rosewood, which also bears the name of *Rhodes-wood*, was imported from Rhodes and some other islands of the Grecian Archipelago. It is hard, heavy, of a dead leaf yellow color, darker in the centre than at the circumference. Its taste is bitter. It is oily, and takes fire easily. Its uses are the same as ordinary rosewood. By distillation these woods yield a volatile oil, which has the odor of rose oil.

Cassia of Perfumers.

A species of locust, originally of the East, and cultivated in Italy, South of France, Algeria, etc. An excellent perfume is extracted from its flowers. It is employed in several preparations, and principally in the alcoholates or extracts of violet.

Cinnamon.

The inner bark of several trees found on the coasts of China and Malabar, in the Island of Ceylon, etc.

There are two varieties especially known to the trade—

1. *Aromatic cinnamon*, from the *laurus cassia*, is coarse and less esteemed than

2. *Ceylon cinnamon*, the product of the *cassia zeylonicum.*

Cinnamon is the inner bark of the branches. There are three qualities of cinnamon, viz., the fine, the middle, and the common. It has been generally ascertained that it is the sound bark of the trunks of the tree cultivated in Ceylon, and the quality depends on the age of the plant and the size of the trunks from which the bark is taken. Fine cinnamon is obtained from the trunks and branches of the tree when about three or four years old. It must have a reddish-yellow shade at first, a sweet taste, a little acrid, a very sweet and penetrating odor. Its texture is fine. It is very brittle.

The middle quality is thicker than the first, having been obtained from the older or larger branches or trunks of the tree. The inhabitants of Ceylon introduce some in the packages they make with the first quality.

The common cinnamon is obtained from the largest branches or the old trees. It is rough, thick, of a livid yellow color, has an acrid taste, leaving some viscosity on the tongue, of a strong smell similar to that of bed-bugs. By distillation it gives more essential oil than the two other qualities, but the oil is heavier and its odor not so sweet.

The adulterations of cinnamon consist in the substitution of other barks more or less analogous to it, or by exhausting it of its essential oil by infusing it in alcohol. But these falsifications are easily detected.

Orris Root.

From a plant belonging to the family of the *Irides*. There are several kinds, viz: 1st. The root of the German orris (*oris nostras*), which grows on old walls, is horizontal, rough, covered with a gray epidermis. It is white inside. Fresh, it has a weak odor of violets and an acrid taste. 2d. The root of the orris of Florence (*iris florentina*), is large as the thumb, heavy, has a fine white color, an acrid and bitter taste, and a decided odor of violets. 3d. The root of the orris, or false acarus of the marshes (*acorus palustris*). 4th. The root of the fetid orris (*iris fœtidissima*) has been recommended as an antispasmodic.

Nard.

A plant of the family of the *graminees*, famous in antiquity on account of the aphrodisiac qualities attributed to its odor. It is in the root that resides the perfume; is used sometimes in perfumery.

Cyperus Odoratus.

This root, like the orris, has an agreeable odor of violets, but weaker and of less duration. Perfumers macerate it in vinegar, and, after drying it in an oven, reduce it to powder to employ it in different preparations.

Zedoary.

Root of a plant belonging to the family of the *cannacorus.* It comes from China, Malabar, and the Philippines, in small pieces two or three inches long, similar in color to orris root.

Is used in pharmacy and perfumery—in the first as a tonic, in the latter as an agreeable perfume.

Galanga.

Root of a little tree belonging to the family of the *cannacorus*, which grows in the East Indias. Its odor is at the same time strong and sweet. Its taste is pricking. The Chinese prepare from it a very sweet essence, used to perfume the tea of the Emperor and great officers of the court.

Calamus Aromaticus.

The root of the *acorus calamus*, a plant which grows in damp and marshy places in the United States, France, and other countries. This root is a little thicker than the finger. At intervals it presents knots. The body is straight, simple, compressed. The dried rhizome of this plant, commonly called *root*, is employed under the name of *calamus aromaticus*. Its aromatic odor is very agreeable, and of long duration; its consistency is spongy; its fracture is resinoid; its color light yellow. It is used by perfumers and distillers to give to some liquors a perfume of orris and cinnamon.

Catechu.

There are two substances having about the same properties and differing in their origin and some other characteristics; they are *catechu* and *kino*. The only one we shall examine is catechu. For a long time it was considered as an earthy substance called *terra japonica*, because it was principally imported from Japan. We now know that it is a vegetable extractive substance. Catechu exists abundantly in the pericarp of several species of the genus *algarobia* and *acacia;* in the wood of the *acacia catechu*, in the nuts of the *areca catechu*, &c. It is extracted by submitting the parts of the plants which contain it to a long ebullition in water and reducing the liquid by evaporation to two-thirds of its volume. The pasty residuum is dried in the sun.

It has a brown color, is solid, not deliquescent; its density varies from 1.28 to 1.39. It cannot be melted; a strong heat decomposes it. Thrown on incandescent coals it burns without leaving any residuum. Soluble in water, alcohol, vinegar, and wine. Its acrid taste is astringent. It contains tannin. The other proximate principles are an *extractive matter*, *mucilage*, *catechucic acid*, and an *insoluble residuum* of an undetermined nature.

It is used in perfumery to make some preparations to disinfect the breath.

Before using it, the perfumer has to purify it to separate the earth it contains; it is sufficient to dissolve it in boiling water, filter, and evaporate the filtrate to the proper consistency.

Sometimes catechu is adulterated with an argillaceous earth, of a brownish-red color. This mixture is easy to detect; it adheres to the tongue, does not melt in the mouth, is not soluble in wine, weak alcohol, or vinegar, and when calcined leaves a residuum. When adulterated with vegetable juices, it is sufficient to add a little brown chloride of iron to an aqueous solution, a black or violet precipitate is thrown down, instead of the green given by pure catechu. If it contains starch, a few drops of a tincture of iodine in its aqueous solution will give a blue color. If mixed with alum, the aqueous solution treated by ammonia and chloride of barium gives a white precipitate, which is not produced with pure catechu.

Vanilla.

Fruit of the *epidendrum vanilla*, a plant of the family of the orchides, which grows principally in Mexico. It is a bean from three to six inches long, the odor of which is well known. It is collected a short time before ripening, then it is covered with a varnish made from coco or castor oil, so as to prevent the volatilization of the aromatic principle. In the trade it is distinguished by the terms *flat* and *long*.

Sometimes a vanilla is found in commerce which has already been used. By chemical processes the greatest part of the perfume has been extracted to make an essence.

It is much used in confectionery and perfumery. Its odoriferous principles have not been well determined; one is a peculiar essential oil, the other an odoriferous acid similar to cinnamic acid.

Nutmeg (Nux myristica).

Fruit of the aromatic nutmeg, a tree originally from the Moluccas. Nutmeg is composed of three parts, the outside, which is rough, called *browse;* the other, called *mace,* which is the shell of the almond; the third is the part called nut.

After the nutmegs are collected, they are deprived of the browse and exposed to the sun to dry them; lastly, they are dipped in lime-water and barrelled to be exported.

By pressure, a concrete oil or butter, with a very sweet odor, is extracted from the nutmeg; if distilled, a strongly aromatic essential oil is obtained.

SECTION II.

NATURAL ESSENTIAL OILS.

THE odoriferous principles of plants may be divided into three kinds: 1. The essential oils; 2. The camphors, balsams, resins; 3. The volatile ethers, similar to those which give their perfumes to wines and fruits. These principles, according to the plants, exist in flowers, leaves or fruits; sometimes in the trunk and bark, in the woods and roots. Thus mint, thyme, etc., contain this principle in the leaves and stems; rose, jasmine, tuberose, etc., in the petals; cinnamon, in the bark; anis, etc., in the seeds; orris, in the root, etc. etc. The different parts of the same plant sometimes afford different perfumes. Green oranges distilled give a product known by the name of *petit grain;* the flowers submitted to the same distillation give *neroli*, and from the bark the oil of Portugal is extracted.

The dissection of plants and their microscopical examination have made known the fact that the odors of the flowers of the plants had their origin in the sexual apparatus; that the odors from the leaves, trunk and bark are furnished by small vesicles filled with essential oils. The odor of the leaves and trunks is not destroyed by the death of the plants, while that of the flowers disappears generally after the fecundation. Double flowers being sterile, have their odor more lasting. These facts are of the highest importance to the grower of plants for the use of the perfumer.

CHAPTER V.

NATURAL STATE OF ESSENTIAL OILS—THEIR MODE OF FORMATION—THEIR GENERAL PROPERTIES—CLASSIFICATION—ADULTERATIONS.

Natural State—Mode of Formation.

ESSENTIAL oils are the production of the vegetable kingdom, and are considered by botanists as secretions. It is to the presence of essential oils that flowers, leaves, roots, etc., owe the odor they exhale. Some plants, in their natural condition, are without odor; nevertheless, an essential oil may be extracted from them, after grinding the organic tissue — for example, the root of the horse-radish. The oil is not ready formed in it, but its elements pre-exist in an isolated form in peculiar cells. If these cells are broken, the liquids they contain are mixed, a spontaneous fermentation takes place, and the oil with a penetrating odor immediately appears. The intervention of water is necessary; indeed, if the substance is dried, no reaction will take place. These essential oils are the basis of the perfumer's trade.

Natural Oils—General Properties.

Natural oils form a group the properties and chemical nature of which are very variable. They have in common the following characteristics:—

A strong odor similar to that of the plant from which they are extracted, an acrid and burning taste, and the property of being very inflammable and of burning with a fuliginous flame. They are volatile and boil at different temperatures (from 284° to 464°), always over the boiling point of water, but a current of steam at 212° carries them off very easily. On account of this property they have received the very improper name of *volatile oils.* They have no analogy with fatty substances. They are all soluble in ether, alcohol, sulphuret of carbon, oils, and greases; very little soluble in water; but this liquid dissolves enough to receive the odor and taste of the oil.

Their density is not uniform. They are generally lighter than water, but some are heavier. Their color varies between the green, yellow, brown, or red shades. One amongst them is blue (oil of camomile). These colors are not inherent to the oils. A well conducted rectification renders them colorless. Generally, they are liquid at the ordinary temperature; some are concrete, as camphor, or have a buttery consistency, as anis, rose, becoming fluid as soon as they are heated. This property of solidifying is due to an excess of the concrete matter which enters into the composition of a great many oils, and which has been called *stearoptene.* Cold separates it from the fluid part called *eloptene,* as when the oil freezes.

The action of the air colors and thickens these oils, and transforms them into a resinous substance, which does not pass over during the distillation. Light greatly favors this transformation. Instead of a resin, the products of the exudation by the air of the oils of cinnamon, bitter almonds, cumin, are well defined acids—the *cinnamic, benzoic,* and *cuminic acids.*

Chlorine, bromine, and iodine decompose them, taking the place of hydrogen, and converting them into new compounds. Phosphorus and sulphur dissolve in them; but the second especially, when warm, decomposes them and changes their nature.

Concentrated nitric acid attacks them violently, generally with the production of flame and explosions. When diluted, the product of the reaction is similar to that resulting from the action of the oxygen of the air; it is a resin or organic acid—sometimes a mixture of both.

Some oils have the property of forming two combinations with alkalies. The oils of cloves, pimento, mustard, are examples. Others, under the influence of a base, are decomposed into an acid which combines with the alkali and a liquid hydrocarbon which separates. Such are the oils of cumin and valerian.

The tendency to play the part of a base is peculiar to those oils with two elements (carbon and hydrogen—$C_{10}H_8$). By absorbing hydrochloric acid gas they give birth to crystalline combinations, which are called *artificial camphors.*

We see from what precedes that great differences exist between the essential oils in view of their chemical characteristics. Their history will not be complete without describing each separately. They are very complex bodies, always rich in carbon and hydrogen, readily decomposed under the influence of chemical agents into a series of compounds, having for their starting point a real or hypothetical radical which plays a part similar to that of cyanogen, viz: Allyl, $C_{12}H_{10}$; benzole, $C_{14}H_6O_2$; cumenyl, $C_{18}H_{11}$.

Classification.

Viewed according to their elementary composition they are divided into three groups:—

1. Essential oils with two elements, liquid hydrocarburets, isomeric in their composition.

2. Oils with three elements, oxygenized hydrocarburets.

3. Sulphuretted oils without oxygen, but containing sulphur and nitrogen.

The following table exhibits the principal essential oils:—

HYDROCARBURETTED.	OXYGENIZED.	SULPHURETTED.
Oil of lemon,	Oil of bitter almonds,	Oil of mustard,
orange,	cinnamon,	garlic,
juniper,	anise,	horseradish,
turpentine,	mint,	cress,
copaiba,	lavender,	assafœtida.
Eleoptene of roses.	valerian,	
	Stearoptene of roses.	

Falsifications.

Volatile oils are frequently adulterated by the addition of fixed oils, resinous substances, and alcohol.

Fixed oils may be known by their leaving a permanent greasy stain upon paper, while that produced by a volatile oil disappears entirely when exposed to heat.

When the adulterated oil is distilled with water, both resin and fixed oil remain behind.

Alcohol may be detected by the milkiness of the oil when agitated with water, after the liquids have separated, the water occupies more volume and the oil less than before. Various methods have been recommended to detect the presence of alcohol in volatile oils. M. Beral put twelve drops of the suspected oil in a perfectly dry watch-glass, and then added a piece of potassium as large as the head of a pin. If the potassium remains for ten or fifteen minutes in the midst of the liquid, there is either no alcohol present or less than four per cent.; if it disappears in five minutes, the oil contains more than five per cent. of alcohol; if no less than a minute, twenty-five per cent. or more. M. Borsarelli introduces small pieces of chloride of calcium, well dried and perfectly free from dust, into a small cylindrical tube, closed at one end, and about two-thirds filled with the oil to be examined, and heats the tube to 212°, occasionally shaking it. If there be a considerable proportion of alcohol, the chloride is entirely dissolved, forming a solution which sinks to the bottom of the tube; if only a very small quantity, the pieces lose their form and collect at the bottom in a white adhering mass; if none at all, they remain unchanged. Bernoulli adds dry acetate of potash to the oil: if alcohol be present, the salt is dissolved, forming a solution from which the volatile oil separates; if the oil be free from alcohol, the salt remains dry therein.

Wittstein, who speaks highly of this test, has suggested the following mode of applying it as the best: In a dry test-tube, half an inch in diameter and five or six inches long, put not more than eight grains of powdered dry acetate of potash, then fill the tube two-thirds full of the volatile oil. The contents of the tube must be well stirred with a glass rod, taking care not to allow the salt to rise above the oil; afterwards set aside for a short time. If the salt be found at the bottom of the tube dry, it is evident that the oil contains no spirit. Often instead of the dry salt beneath the oil is found a clear syrupy fluid, which is a solution of the salt in the alcohol with which the oil was mixed. When the oil contains only a little alcohol, a small portion of the solid salt will be found under the syrupy solution. Many oils frequently contain a trace of water, which does not materially interfere with this test, because, although the acetate of potash becomes moist thereby, it still retains its pulverulent form. Oberdoffer places from two to four drachms of the suspected oil in a flat glass plate, in the middle of which is placed a small glass stand, on which a watch-glass with five or ten grains of platinum black is supported, and the whole is covered by a glass bell open at the top. In the course of a few minutes, oil containing alcohol begins to redden litmus paper, which in the space of a quarter or half an hour is completely accomplished, the eliminated vapors of acetic acid are deposited in the interior of the glass bell, if the alcohol is present in sufficient quantity, and can be recognized distinctly by its odor. To remove all doubt he washes the platinum black with a little water, filters, saturates the filtrate carefully with potash, and adds neutral chloride of iron, by which the characteristic odor of acetate of iron is obtained; and, after boiling, the fluid becomes decolorized and the hydrated oxide of iron is precipitated. From a series of experiments he concludes that it is possible in this way to detect the presence of one or two per cent. of alcohol, and that with five per cent. the odor is sufficient with most oils to prove the admixture of alcohol.

It is frequently the case that essential oils of small value are mixed with the more costly. These may be detected by their taste, odor, and specific gravity. Oil of turpentine, which is a common adulteration, may be known by remaining partly undissolved when the oil is treated with three or four times its volume of alcohol. Turpentine may be detected more easily by a very simple experiment, based on the peculiar action of damp air on spirits of turpentine. If with the mouth we blow in a bottle three-quarters full of turpentine quietly enough not to disturb the liquid, a little dampness condenses on the oil, and white lines are formed which like clouds descend in the liquid. By repeating this experiment on pure lavender or mint oils, the moisture does not descend in the form of clouds, but as beads; while, if mixed with turpentine, it behaves as turpentine itself. This phenomenon is produced with five per cent. of oil of turpentine, and very few oils in the market will resist that test.

CHAPTER VI.

EXTRACTION OF ESSENTIAL OILS—BY DISTILLATION—DISTILLATION OF LIGHT OILS—DISTILLATION OF HEAVY OILS—DISTILLATION BY REACTION—BY IMPREGNATION—BY EXPRESSION.

THE processes employed to extract from plants the essential oil they contain are: 1. *The distillation of the plants* with natural water or with salt water; 2. By impregnation with fatty bodies; 3. By pressure.

Distillation.

Distillation is generally effected in an alembic, the description of which is given in Chapter IV.

The distillation may be made by three different processes.

1. With a *naked fire*, that is, when the cucurbit is placed directly on the fire itself.

2. Over a *water bath*, or *sand bath*, or *oil bath*—when the cucurbit is placed in a kettle containing water or oil in a boiling state, or in sand heated by a furnace. In these three cases, the fire acts only indirectly on the cucurbit, and the degree of heat is constantly the same.

3. *By steam.* This third method of distillation

is made by means of a curved pipe, which conducts the steam from a boiler into the alembic.

During distillation over a naked fire, the substances to be distilled are disposed on a metallic diaphragm, or on a simple bed of straw on the bottom of the cucurbit, to isolate the material from the bottom and prevent its burning.

Adapt the head, then the worm, and the receiver. Begin to heat, and raise the temperature to 212°. The distillation soon begins. When ordinary water is used, all the salts it contains remain at the bottom of the cucurbit, while the pure water volatilizes and condenses in the worm, and thence runs into the receiver.

The essential oils are divided into *light oils* and *heavy oils.* The first floats on the water of the receiver; the second, heavier than water, falls to the bottom.

DISTILLATION OF LIGHT ESSENTIAL OILS.

Oil of Orange Flower.

Fresh orange flowers .	4 pounds.
Pure water	12 "

Introduce the flowers into a bag of metallic cloth, place this bag in the cucurbit containing the necessary quantity of water, adapt the head and the refrigerator, heat and distil until no more water and oil pass over. Decant the oil floating on the surface of the water, and filter if necessary. During the operation, the refrigerator must be kept very cool. The cooler it is, the better the product. Some macerate the flowers for twenty-four hours in salt water, and then distil.

The following essential oils may be obtained in the same manner:—

Sweet Basil,	Sage,	Bergamot,
Hyssop,	Serpolet,	Bitter Orange,
Lavender,	Thyme,	Cedrat,
Marjoram,	Anis,	Lemon,
Marruba,	Caraway,	Small Orange,
Melissa,	Coriander,	Orange,
Mint,	Cumin,	Wormwood,
Origanum,	Fennel,	Camomile, etc.
Rosemary,		

By using the Florentine receiver the essential oil will run off by a small pipe, which thus does away with the decanting process.

DISTILLATION OF THE HEAVY ESSENTIAL OILS.

Oil of Cloves.

Coarsely powdered cloves .	5 pounds.
Water	10 "
Salt	1 pound.

Macerate forty-eight hours, and distil until the product is no longer milky. Allow the essential oil to deposit; decant the water, which is poured back into the alembic, and distil a second time. This operation is repeated two or three times to extract all the oil. Ten days after, the oil is filtered to clarify and deprive it of all foreign matters.

The oils of cinnamon, Rhodium-wood, sandal, calamus, aloes, etc. etc., are obtained in the same manner.

DISTILLATION BY REACTION.

Essential Oil of Bitter Almonds.

Ground cake of bitter almonds . 2 pounds.
Cold water . . a sufficient quantity.

Mix the cake in the water so as to make a light paste, which is introduced into the cucurbit and permitted to macerate for twenty-four hours. After this time, distil by means of steam. Continue the distillation until it has passed over four pounds; separate the oil, which is heavier than water; put back the water in the alembic and distil anew, and continue the operation in the same manner until no more oil passes over.

The essential oil of mustard is obtained by the same process.

Process by Impregnation of Fatty Bodies.

There are flowers with fugitive odors, such as jonquil, violet, jasmine, &c., the perfume of which is very difficult to fix. The ordinary distillation gives a weak product; that with alcohol is not more satisfactory. They can be fixed only by combining them with a fixed oil, and distilling the latter with alcohol. In treating of the *extracts of flowers* we shall enter more into the details of this process.

Process by Expression.

Fruits with odoriferous rinds, and particularly the orange, cedrat, bergamot, lemon, &c., may be pressed to extract their essential oils. By this process the oils are finer and sweeter. The method of operating is the following: Remove the outer skin of the rinds by grating, without touching the white, and put them into a porcelain jar. When all the *zestes* are ready, put them in a bag of common cloth, and place them under a press, which is turned slowly, so as to produce a moderate pressure without tearing the bag. The oil thus obtained is poured into a jar with a little alum, to help the precipitation of the mucilage, and the next day the oil is decanted. Some perfumers, instead of separating the *zestes*, scrape the rind, but this process takes some of the white, and gives an oil of inferior quality. Others cut the rind into pieces and throw them into tepid water, in which they are left a few hours; they then introduce the mass into an alembic, and distil over a water bath.

There is a method of distilling without the alembic, practised in some Eastern countries, which we shall now describe.

1. A large vessel, having the form of a thimble,

which is half filled with roses, or some other flowers.

2. A smaller vessel, with a large mouth, placed on a stand inside of the larger one. The top of this small vessel rises about one inch above the flowers.

3. A hollow cone of sheet iron, the base of which hermetically closes the opening of the large vessel, and the point of which descends just above the middle of the smaller. The sheet-iron cone is filled with pieces of ice. The apparatus, thus arranged, is put in a sand bath and heated; the oil crystallizes, is cooled by the ice in the cone, condenses, and falls in drops into the small vessel. The operation completed, the small vessel is sunken, and the oil separated from the water.

The quality and quantity of the oils obtained depend on many contingencies—on the mode of operation, on the state of maturity or conservation of the plants, climate, the localities they come from. Vegetables growing in arid, mountainous soils, have the preference. It is in the morning that flowers should be gathered and immediately distilled; plants which are left gathered several days grow warm, begin to ferment, and the essential oil they yield is of a poor quality.

Essential oils must be kept in bottles hermetically sealed, covered with black or blue paper, and placed in a cool place. Blue glass bottles will be the best to preserve essential oils from the action of light and the oxygen of the air.

The following table gives the amount of essential oil obtained from 100 pounds of material.

Names.	100 lbs. gave essential oils	Names.	100 lbs. gave essential oils
Bitter almonds .	3 ounces	Cherry laurel .	2 ounces
Spike	8 "	Lavender . . .	10½ "
Badian . . .	18 "	Melisse . . .	2 "
Sweet basil . .	7 "	Peppermint . .	4 "
Herb benne . .	1 ounce	Orange . . .	4 "
Bergamot. . .	2½ ounces	Green orange .	4½ "
Garden balsam .	2 "	Origanum. . .	3 dr'ms
Cinnamon. . .	1½ "	Rosemary . .	3½ ozs.
Caraway . . .	50 "	Sandal. . . .	3½ "
Cedrat. . . .	1½ "	Wild thyme . .	3½ "
Citronella. . .	1 ounce	Thyme. . . .	3 "
Lemon. . . .	1 "	Vervain . . .	.3 "
Cloves	66 ounces	Fennel . . .	6 "
Hyssop . . .	5½ "		

CHAPTER VII.

ESSENTIAL OILS THE MOST USED IN PERFUMERY.

Oil of Roses.—This is one of the most important essential oils; it is obtained simply by distilling the roses with water.

The *otto* or *attar* of rose of commerce is derived from the *rosa centifolia provincialis.* Extensive farms exist at Broussa, at Uslak (Turkey in Asia), also at Ghazepore in India. In a good season the rose farms of the Balkan yield 75,000 ounces, but in bad seasons only 20,000 to 30,000 ounces. It requires at least 16,000 flowers to yield one ounce of otto.

The otto from different districts slightly varies in odor; many places furnish an otto which solidifies more readily than others, and therefore this is not a sure guide of purity, though many so consider it. The French otto is richer in stearopten than the Turkish, one ounce and a half will crystallize in one gallon of spirit at the same temperature that is required for three ounces of the best Turkish otto.

Its color is slightly yellow, with a very sweet odor; lighter than water, solid at the temperature of 50° to 54°. According to the experiments of De Saussure, it is formed of two oils, one solid and the other liquid. They can be separated by treating them with rectified alcohol at the temperature of 32°, which dissolves all the liquid, and only traces of the solid.

There are six modifications of essence of rose for the handkerchief. They are—the spirit of treble rose, essence of white rose, essence of tea rose, essence of moss rose, twin rose, and Chinese rose. The following are the recipes for their formation:—

Treble Spirit of Rose.

Rectified alcohol	1 gallon.
Otto of rose	3 ounces.

Twin Rose.

Rose pomade	8 pounds.
Spirit at 75°	1 gallon.
Otto of rose	1½ ounce.

Essence of Moss Rose.

Spirituous extract from rose pomatum	1 quart.
Treble spirit of rose . . .	1 pint.
Extract fleur d'orange pomatum	1 "
ambergris . . .	½ "
musk	4 ounces.

Essence of White Rose.

Spirit of rose from pomatum	.	1 quart.
treble	. . .	1 "
violet	. . .	1 "
Extract of jasmin	. . .	1 pint.
patchouly	. . .	½ "

Essence of Tea Rose.

Esprit de rose pomade	. .	1 pint.
treble	. . . .	1 "
Extract of rose-leaf geranium	.	1 "
sandal-wood	. .	½ "
neroli	. . .	¼ "
orris	. . . .	¼ "

Chinese Yellow Rose.

Esprit de rose triple	. . .	2 pints.
tuberose	. . .	2 "
tonquin	. . .	¼ pint.
vervain	. . .	¼ "

The otto of rose is always very costly, and consequently is often adulterated. The falsifications are easily detected, and if it does not solidify at 50°, it may be considered as adulterated.

Oil of Orange Flower.—Two distinct odors can be obtained from the orange blossom, varying according to the methods of extraction.

When orange flowers are treated by maceration, the orange flower pomatum is obtained. It requires sixteen pounds of blossom to enflower two pounds of grease divided over thirty-two infusions, that is, half a pound of flowers to every two pounds of fat for each maceration.

By macerating the pomatum in rectified spirits the extract of orange flower is obtained. In this state its odor resembles the original so much that with closed eyes the best judge cannot distinguish the extract from the flower.

When orange flowers are distilled with water the otto is obtained, which is commercially known by the name of *neroli*. The finest is obtained from the *citrus aurantium*, and is called neroli petale. The next quality (neroli bigarrade) is obtained from the *citrus bigaradia* ; a second quality, which is considered inferior to the above, is the neroli petit grain, obtained by distilling the leaves and unripe fruit of the different species of the *citrus*.

Its color varies from a reddish-yellow to a dark red; it is very fluid. It is sometimes adulterated with alcohol, or oil of small oranges.

Oil of Orange.—Under the title *neroli* we have already spoken of the odoriferous principle of the orange blossom. We have now to speak of what is known in the market as oil of orange.

The otto of orange peel is procured by expression and by distillation. The peel is rasped in order to crush the little vessels that contain the oil. It has many uses in perfumery, it is the leading ingredient of what is sold as *eau de Portugal*, which may be prepared as follows:—

Lisbon Water.

Rectified spirit at 75°	. .	1 gallon.
Otto of orange peel	. .	4 ounces.
lemon zest	. .	2 "
rose	. . . .	¼ ounce.

Eau de Portugal.

Rectified spirit at 75°	. .	1 gallon.
Ess. oil of orange peel	. .	8 ounces.
lemon zest	. .	2 "
bergamot	. .	1 ounce.
otto of rose	. .	¼ "

Oil of Lemon.—This fine perfume is extracted from the *citrus limonum* by expression and also by distillation. The oil obtained by expression has a much finer odor and a more intense lemon smell than the distilled product.

The otto of lemon found in the market comes principally from Messina, where there are hundreds of acres of lemon groves.

Ordinary lemon oil weighs fourteen ounces per pint. It has a yellowish color, soluble in all proportions in pure alcohol. It is rapidly oxidized when in contact with the air and exposed to light. On account of this rapid oxidization it should not be used for perfuming greases, as it assists all fats to become rancid. In the manufacture of other compound perfumes, it should be dissolved in spirit in the proportion of six to eight ounces of oil to one gallon of spirit.

Oil of Lavender.—Lavender is grown to an enormous extent at Mitcham, in Surrey, England, and at Hitchin, in Hertfordshire, which are the places of production in a commercial point of view. Very large quantities are also grown in France, which is remarkably good, but by their fine odor the British products realize in the market four times the price of that of continental growth. Half a hundred weight of good lavender flowers yields by distillation from fourteen to sixteen ounces of essential oil. The number of lavender plants upon an acre of ground would be about 3547, that is, if planted one yard apart and four feet between the rows. An acre would yield from six to seven quarts of oil.

There are two methods of making the essence of lavender: by distilling a mixture of essential oil of lavender and rectified spirit; 2d, by merely mixing the oil and the spirit together. The latter process yields the finest quality.

Smyth's Lavender.

To produce a very fine distillate, take—

Otto of English lavender .	4 ounces.
Rectified alcohol at 75° .	5 pints.
Rose water . . .	1 pint.

Mix and distil 5 pints.

Essence of Lavender.

Otto of lavender . . .	6 ounces.
Rectified alcohol . .	1 gallon.

Mix.

Pure oil of lavender should have a specific gravity from 0.876 to 0.880, and be completely soluble in five parts of alcohol. A greater specific gravity shows that it is mixed with oil of spike, and a less solubility that it contains turpentine.

Oil of Rosemary.—By distilling the *rosmarinus officinalis*, a thin, limpid otto is obtained, having the characteristic odor of the plant, which is more aromatic than sweet. One hundred weight of the fresh herb yields about twenty-four ounces of oil. It is limpid, white, or yellowish; is lighter than water; its specific gravity = 0.91, and only 0.89 when carefully rectified.

Otto of rosemary is extensively used in perfumery, especially in combination with other ottoes for scenting soaps. It is the leading ingredient of the Hungary water, which is thus made:—

Hungary Water.

Pure alcohol at 95° . . .	1 gallon.
Otto of Hungarian rosemary	2 ounces.
lemon peel . . .	1 ounce.
melissa	1 "
mint	½ drachm.
spirit of rose . . .	1 pint.
Extract of fleur d'orange .	1 "

Oil of Rhodium Wood.—When rose-wood (*convolvulus scoparius*) is distilled, a sweet-smelling oil is obtained, resembling in fragrance the odor of the rose, and hence its name. At one time the distillates from rose-wood, and from the canary rose-wood (*geniata canariensis*) were principally used for the adulteration of real otto of roses; but as geranium oil answers better, the oil of rhodium has fallen into disuse.

Oil of Geranium.—The leaves of the rose-leaf geranium (*pelargonium odoratissimum*) yield by distillation a very agreeable rose-smelling otto, so much resembling that of rose that it is extensively used to adulterate that costly substance. One hundred pounds of leaves give two ounces of oil. Some samples are greenish colored, others nearly white; that with a brownish tint is the best.

Oil of Cedrat.—This is obtained from the rind of the citron fruit (*citrus medica*) both by distillation and expression. It has a beautiful lemony odor. It is principally used in the manufacture of essences for handkerchiefs.

Oil of Bergamot.—This is obtained from the *citrus bergamia* by expression from the peel of the fruit. One hundred fruits will yield about three ounces of the otto. When new and good it has a greenish-yellow tint, but loses its greenness by age, and oxidizes rapidly under the influence of the air. It is extensively used in perfumery.

Oil of Peppermint.—There are several plants which yield fragrant oils when distilled with steam; amongst them peppermint holds a high place. About three thousand acres of it are under cultivation, viz., one thousand in New York and Ohio, and two thousand in St. Joseph County, Michigan. It is used exclusively for its oil, about seven pounds of which is the average yield for one acre.

The apparatus for distilling peppermint consists of a boiler for raising steam, a wooden still, a cooler, and a receiver. The plants are packed in the still and trampled down. When a full charge is ready the lid of the still is put on, and steam admitted at the bottom. When the temperature is raised to 212° the oil passes over with the steam, and condenses in the receiver.

This oil is more used in confectionery than perfumery.

Oil of Mint.—All the *menthida* yield fragrant ottoes by distillation. The otto of the spearmint (*M. viridis*) is very powerful, and valuable for perfuming soap. It is extensively used for mouth-washes and dental liquids.

Oil of Wintergreen.—This is obtained by distilling the leaves of the *gaultheria procumbens.* When the plant is distilled, at first an oil passes over, which consists of $C_{10}H_8$, but when the temperature reaches 464° the pure oil distils. It is a colorless liquid, with an agreeable aromatic odor and taste; it dissolves slightly in water; but in all proportions in alcohol and ether. It boils between 411° and 435°, and its specific gravity = 1.173. Its formula is $C_{16}H_8O_6$.

A very nice handkerchief perfume is prepared upon the strength of the name of this odorous plant. It is called

Iceland Wintergreen.

Esprit de rose	1	pint.
Essence of lavender	4	ounces.
Extract of neroli	8	"
vanilla	4	"
vitivert	4	"
cassia	8	"
ambergris	4	"

Oil of Sandal.—This oil is extracted from the sandal-wood (*santalum album*) by distillation. One hundred weight of wood will yield thirty ounces of otto.

It is very heavy, and has a dark straw color. When dissolved in spirit, it enters into the composition of a great many of the old fashioned bouquets. Perfumers use the following formula to make what is called

Extract de Bois de Santal.

Rectified alcohol	7	pints.
Spirits of roses	1	pint.
Ess. oil of sandal	3	ounces.

Oil of Cinnamon.—That known by the name of *oil of Ceylon* is extracted from the *laurus cinnamomum;* another, called *oil of China, oil of cassia,* is extracted from the *laurus cassia.* Both have a light yellow color, an agreeable, sweet and aromatic taste.

Oil of Cloves.—The otto of cloves is obtained by expression from the fresh flower buds of the clove plant (*caryophyllus aromaticus*), but the usual method of procuring it is by distillation. It is extensively used in perfumery with greases, soap, and spirits.

Oil of Allspice is obtained by distilling the dry fruit, before it is quite ripe, of the *Eugenia pimenta* and *myrtus pimento* with water. It is not much used in perfumery, and then only in combination with other spices for scenting soaps.

Oil of Sage is extracted from the leaves and flowers of the plant of that name (*salvia officinalis*). It is yellowish, with a bitter taste, and the penetrating odor of sage.

Oil of Thyme.—Obtained by distillation of the tops of the thyme (*thymus vulgaris*). It has a light yellow color, very odoriferous, hot and acrid to the taste. By settling, it deposits cubic crystals having the odor of thyme, insoluble in water, soluble in alcohol. Oil of thyme is used as perfume in some liquors and cosmetic preparations.

Oil of Anise is obtained by the distillation of the seeds of the plant *pimpinella anisum.* This oil congeals at about 50° F. It is frequently adulterated with a little spermaceti. As the oil of aniseed is quite soluble in alcohol, and the spermaceti is not, the fraud is easily detected.

This perfume is well adapted for mixing with soap and for scenting pomatums, but does not do nicely in compounds for handkerchiefs.

Melissa Oil.—Obtained by distilling the leaves of the *melissa officinalis* with water; comes from the still-tap with the condensed steam. It is very little used in perfumery.

Tuberose Oil, one of the sweetest perfumes, is obtained by *enfleurage* from the tuberose flower. It is much in demand by perfumers for compounding sweet essences. It requires six pounds of flowers to perfume two pounds of grease.

To obtain the extract of tuberose, eight pounds of tuberose pomatum cut very fine are placed in one gallon of rectified alcohol. After standing three or four weeks, with frequent agitation, it is drawn off, strained through a cloth, and the product ready for sale.

This essence is exceedingly volatile, and if sold in its pure state, quickly flies off. It is therefore necessary to add some fixing ingredients, and for this purpose it is best to use an ounce of tincture of storax or half an ounce of extract of vanilla to every pint of tuberose.

Violet Oil is obtained from the *viola odorata*. It is a fugacious oil. For commercial purposes, the odor of violets is procured in combination with spirit, oil, or suet, proceeding to the methods described to obtain the aroma of some other flowers, such as cassie, jasmine, etc., namely, by maceration or enfleurage, the former method being adopted first, followed by enfleurage; and, when essence is required, digesting the pomade in rectified alcohol.

Good essence of violet is of a beautiful green color, and though of a rich deep tint, does not stain white fabrics, and its odor is perfectly natural.

The essence of violets is thus made: Take from six to eight pounds of violet pomade, chip it up fine, and place it in one gallon of rectified alcohol, allow it to digest three weeks or a month, strain, and to every pint add three ounces of tincture of orris root and three ounces spirit of cassia.

A good imitation essence of violet is prepared thus:—

Spirituous extract of cassia pomade .	1 pint.
Esprit de rose, from pomade . .	8 ounces.
Tincture of orris	8 "
Spirituous extract of tuberose pomade	8 "
Otto of almonds	3 drops.

Filter.

Oil of Jonquil.—The scent of jonquil is very fine for perfumery purposes; it is prepared in the same manner as jasmine. An imitation extract of jonquil is prepared as follows:—

Spirituous extract of jasmine pomade	1	pint.
tuberose . .	1	"
orange flower .	8	ounces.
Extract of vanilla	2	"

True Extract of Jonquil.

Jonquil pomade	8	pounds.
Alcohol at 75°	1	gallon.

Macerate one month.

Oil of Heliotrope is obtained, either by maceration or enfleurage with clarified fat, from the flowers of *heliotropium peruvianum* or *H. grandiflorum.* It is not much used now in perfumery. The odor of heliotrope resembles a mixture of almonds and vanilla, and is well imitated thus:—

Spirituous extract of vanilla . .	8	ounces.
rose pomatum .	4	"
orange flower .	2	"
ambergris . .	1	ounce.
Essential oil of almonds . . .	5	drops.

Oil of Jasmine.—This flower is one of the most esteemed by the perfumer. Its odor is delicate and sweet. When the flowers of the *jasminum odoratissimum* are distilled, repeatedly using the water on fresh flowers, the essential oil is obtained. It is exceedingly rare on account of the cost of production.

The method of obtaining the odor is by enfleurage, as we have described. It requires six pounds of flowers to perfume two pounds of grease.

Oils strongly impregnated with the fragrant perfumes are also prepared much in the same way. Cotton cloths previously steeped in olive oil are covered with the flowers, which is repeated several times, finally the cloths are squeezed under a press. The oil thus produced is the *huile antique au jasmin.*

The extract of jasmine is prepared by treating two pounds of pomade by one quart of spirit.

The extract of jasmine is extensively used in perfumery.

Oil of Lilac.—The fragrance of this flower is well known. The oil is obtained either by maceration or enfleurage. The odor so much resembles tuberose as to be frequently used to adulterate the latter.

A beautiful imitation is thus made:—

Spirituous extract from tuberose pomade	1 pint.
Spirituous extract from orange-flower pomade	4 ounces.
Otto of almonds	3 drops.
Extract of civet	4 drachms.

Oil of Lily.—This oil is prepared by infusion, but to obtain anything like its fragrance the operation must be repeated a dozen times with the same oil, using fresh flowers. The oil being shaken with an equal quantity of spirit gives up its odor to the alcohol. An artificial extract of lily is thus made:—

Extract of	tuberose	8 ounces.
	jasmine	1 ounce.
	fleur d'orange	2 ounces.
	vanilla	3 "
	cassia	5 "
	rose	4 "
Oil of almonds		3 drops.

Macerate for one month, and it is ready for sale.

Oil of Magnolia.—The perfume of the flower is superb, but of very little use, on account of the large size of the blossoms and their scarcity. An imitation of this oil is thus made:—

Spirituous extract of orange-flower pomatum	1 pint.
Spirituous extract of rose pomatum	2 pints.
Spirituous extract of tuberose pomatum	8 ounces.
Spirituous extract of violet pomatum	8 "
Otto of citron zest	3 drachms.
almonds	10 drops.

Oil of Myrtle.—A very fragrant oil may be obtained by distilling the leaves of the common myrtle. The demand for this essence is limited, and that sold under the name is an imitation thus made:—

Extract of vanilla	8	ounces.
roses	16	"
fleur d'orange	8	"
tuberose	8	"
jasmine	2	"

Mix, let it stand fifteen days, and bottle.

Oil of Sweet-brier exists in the perfumers' shops only by name, for it does not pay for the labor of collecting. That sold under the name is an imitation thus prepared:—

Spirituous extract of rose pomatum	1	pint.
cassia	4	ounces.
fleur d'orange	4	"
Esprit de rose	4	"
Oil de neroli	½	drachm.
Oil of verbena	½	"

Oil of Cassia is one of those fine odors which enter into the composition of the best bouquets. It is procured by maceration from the *acacia farnesiana*. It requires two pounds of flowers to perfume one pound of grease. The oil is prepared in the same manner, only substituting olive oil by suet.

The extract is prepared by treating six pounds of pomade by one gallon of rectified spirit. After a maceration of three or four weeks, it is fit to draw off, and, if good, has a beautiful olive green color and the rich smell of cassia blossoms.

Cedar Oil.—Cedar wood, when distilled, yields

an essential oil that is exceedingly fragrant, and which is used extensively for scenting cold cream soap. The following is the formula for the *Lebanon cedar wood* for the handkerchief:—

Otto of cedar	. . .	1 ounce.
Rectified spirit	. . .	16 ounces.
Esprit de rose triple	. .	4 "

Oil of Citronella.—Under this name there is an oil in the market, chiefly from Ceylon. It is procured by distilling the leaves of the *andropogon schœnanthus*, which grows wild in Ceylon. Citronella being cheap, is extensively used for perfuming soaps. The honey soap is a fine yellow soap perfumed with this oil.

Oil of Verbena, or Vervain.—Obtained, by distillation with water, of the leaves of the *aloysia citriodora*, but on account of its high price is scarcely used; but is most successfully imitated by mixing the oil of lemon grass (*andropogon nardus*) with rectified alcohol. The following is a good form for making the *extract of verbena:*—

Rectified alcohol	. .	1 pint.
Oil of lemon grass	. .	3 drachms.
lemon peel	. .	2 ounces.
Orange peel	. .	½ ounce.

Another mixture of this kind, but of finer quality, is prepared thus (it is sold under the name of *extrait de verveine*):—

Rectified spirit . . .	1	pint.
Oil of orange peel . .	1	ounce.
lemon peel . .	2	ounces.
citron zest . .	1	drachm.
lemon grass . .	2½	drachms.
Extrait de fleur d'orange .	7	ounces.
tuberose . .	7	"
Esprit de rose . . .	8	"

This mixture is one of the most elegant perfumes for the handkerchief.

Oil of Vitivert is prepared by distillation from the kus-kus, the rhizome of an Indian grass. It is a very agreeable oil, which very much resembles otto of sandal.

The essence of vitivert of the shops is prepared by steeping, for fifteen days, four pounds of dried vitivert in one gallon of rectified alcohol. It is also made by dissolving two ounces of otto in one gallon of spirit.

Either the extract, essence, or tincture of vitivert enters into the composition of many bouquets for the handkerchief.

Volkameria. — An exquisite perfume is sold under this name, supposed to be derived from the *volkameria inermis*—a native of India, and very little known even by botanists. What is sold under the name of essence of volkameria is thus composed:—

Esprit de violette	. .	1 pint.
tubereuse	. .	1 "
jasmin	. .	¼ "
rose	. . .	½ "
Essence de musc	. . .	2 ounces.

Wallflower.—Exquisite as is the odor of this flower, it is not used in perfumery, while its perfume may be obtained in the same manner as that of heliotrope and jasmine. An imitation of essence of wallflower may be thus prepared:—

Extrait de fleur d'orange	.	1 pint.
vanille	. .	8 ounces.
Esprit de rose	. . .	1 pint.
Extract of orris	. . .	8 ounces.
cassie	. .	8 "
Ess. oil of almonds	. .	5 drops.

Macerate two or three weeks, and put in bottle.

Imitation of Oil of Honeysuckle.

Spirituous extract of rose pomatum	.	1 pint.
violet	. .	1 "
tuberose	. .	1 "
Extract of vanilla	. . . . .	4 ounces.
tolu	. . . . .	4 "
Otto neroli	. . . . . .	10 drops.
" almonds	. . . . .	5 "

Mix.

Artificial Extract of Narcissus.

Extract of tuberose . .	3 pints.
jonquil . .	2 "
storax . .	4 ounces.
tolu . . .	4 "

Mix.

Extract of Patchouly.

Rectified alcohol . .	1 gallon.
Otto of patchouly. . .	1¼ ounce.
rose . . .	¼ "

Essence of Ambergris.

Spirit	1 gallon.
Ambergris	3 ounces.

Let it stand one month.

Extrait d'Ambre.

Esprit de rose triple . .	½ pint.
Extract of ambergris . .	1 "
Essence of musk . .	¼ "
Extract of vanilla . .	2 ounces.

Extract of Musk.

Musk	2 ounces.
Rectified alcohol . . .	1 gallon.

Let it stand one month, and draw off.

Extrait de Musc.

Extract of musk (as above) .	1 pint.
ambergris . .	8 ounces.
rose triple . .	4 "

Mix, and filter.

SECTION III.

ARTIFICIAL ESSENTIAL OILS.

THE study of the numerous compounds of organic chemistry, especially the ethers derived from alcohol and potato oil, has produced, of late, an industrial result as curious as interesting, in view of its various applications. Indeed, while chemical analysis found, in the composition of some perfumes, real organic ethers, synthesis, on the other hand, realizing the direct production of these same ethers, taught the chemist to prepare them in such a state of purity that it was easy to confound them, by their physical properties, with the natural perfumes. From this double discovery has risen, little by little, an industry which, in a short time, has acquired in France, England, and Germany, considerable importance. Its object is to manufacture liquids, often complex in their composition, which, dissolved in a certain quantity of pure alcohol, are known by the name of *artificial oils*. Compounds may also be prepared which communicate to ordinary alcohol the odor, but not the qualities, of brandy, whiskey, etc.; and others, which are much used in confectionery, possess the taste of pineapple, strawberry, pear, apple, &c. We must also consider, but only in a commercial point of view, nitrobenzine as an artificial oil. This product, very different in its chemical composition from those we have spoken of, is in great demand by perfumers, who use it instead of oil of bitter almonds to perfume soaps.

The preparation of these products is kept secret by manufacturers; however, we can give some information on the subject which will guide the reader who would study the subject.

CHAPTER VIII.

ARTIFICIAL OILS—OIL OF BRANDY AND WINE—OILS OF RUM — STRAWBERRY — PINEAPPLE—PEAR— APPLE —APRICOT —MELON —QUINCE—CUCUMBERS—LEMON—NITRO-BENZINE—TABLE.

Oil of Brandy and Wine.

THE substance used under this name is a complex mixture of several ethers of the ethylic series, but the odoriferous qualities appear to be due apparently to pelargonic ether. Two methods may be used to prepare it; the first gives pelargonic ether nearly pure—the other gives a mixture of very variable composition and of inferior quality.

In the first case, the oil furnished by the distillation of the *ruta graveolens*, and known in the trade by the name of oil of rue, is the starting point of the operation. Treated by nitrid acid, this oil is transformed into pelargonic acid, which is easily etherefied. The preparation is then divided into two distinct phases.

Introduce into a large retort equal parts of oil of rue and nitric acid diluted with its volume of water. Then heat gently. The reaction is not long to begin; red vapors are abundantly disengaged. As soon as this effect is manifested, the heat is stopped. When the disengagement of red vapors and the attack of the oil have diminished in intensity, cause the contents of the retort to boil, and continue until no more red vapors are disengaged. Collect the oil which floats on the surface of the acid. It is impure pelargonic acid, formed by the oxidation of the oil. Before transforming this acid into ether, it is necessary to purify it; for this purpose treat the crude pelargonic acid by a solution of potash, which dissolves it, leaving a very bitter oil in an insoluble state. The pelargonate of potash, afterwards decomposed by adding little by little sulphuric acid until saturated, furnishes pelargonic acid, which, being washed with water, is sufficiently pure.

To transform pelargonic acid into ether, dissolve it in concentrated alcohol, and pass through the solution a current of dry hydrochloric acid gas. The liquor becomes muddy, and some oily drops are seen to ascend to the surface, which form a bed of pelargonic ether, colorless or slightly yellowish, with an odor similar to that of butyric, capric, etc. ethers.

In the second case, it is by the oxidation of fatty acids that we obtain ethers having the odor of wine and brandy. When neutral or fatty acid bodies are submitted to the action of concentrated nitric acid, two kinds of products are formed—non-volatile acids, such as pimelic, adipic, lauric, etc., acids which remain in solution—and volatile acids which distil over, the principal of which are the butyric, valerianic, capric, caproic, caprylic, œnanthylic, etc.; and amongst them also figure the pelargonic acid.

This reaction is utilized in the following manner: Take a fatty body, solid or liquid—oleic acid is one of those which succeeds the best; place it within eight or ten times its volume of concentrated nitric acid in a retort, as indicated above; then heat with the same precautions. The more concentrated the acid the larger will be the proportion of pelargonic acid obtained. The operation is continued until all the fat has disappeared. The product contained in the receiver is composed of nitric acid and of an oily bed of volatile acids, which are washed two or three times with water and transformed into ethers, in the same manner as for pelargonic acid.

Sometimes, also, to aromatize alcohol, they use the product obtained by etherefying cocinic acid extracted from coco oil. To prepare it, saponify coco oil by a lye of potash, of a density of about 1.12. Decompose this soap by hydrochloric acid, and the soft product thus obtained is pressed to separate the oleic acid. The cocinic acid furnished by the pressure is dissolved in alcohol, and treated while warm by a current of dry hydrochloric acid gas. A slightly yellowish liquid is thus obtained; it has a penetrating odor; it is washed with water, then with a weak solution of carbonate of soda; it is cocinic ether nearly pure.

These different products are met in commerce only in solution in alcohol, to which they are generally added in the proportion of about ten per cent. It is easy to estimate their richness in artificial oils; indeed, they are all less volatile than alcohol, and by distilling them, and collecting only the products passing between 176° and 185°, all the alcohol is obtained in the receiver, while the oil is left in the retort.

Oil of Rum, Strawberries, Pineapple.

Butyric ether, in the preparation of artificial oils, plays a very important part. When pure, it has the fine odor of the pineapple; and it is easy, by the additional use of vinic and amylic alcohol, to modify that odor and change it into that of strawberries, raspberries, etc. Less pure, and mixed with the ethers which accompany it when extracted from natural fatty bodies, it is successfully used to aromatize rum of bad quality.

Two methods are employed to prepare this compound. The first, which gives a pure product, employs butyric acid obtained by the fermentation of sugar; the second employs directly the compounds obtained by the fermentation of butter. To follow the first method, make a solution of sugar which marks 10°; to this solution add white cheese in the proportion of 10 per cent., and powdered chalk in the proportion of 30 per cent. of the molasses. When the mixture is complete, submit it to a temperature of 77° to 86°. A slow fermentation soon begins in the mass, and when, after six weeks, all disengagement of gas has ceased, it is finished. Then add to the mixture its volume of cold water and crystallized carbonate of soda in the proportion of 130 per cent. of the weight of the sugar. Further to separate the carbonate of lime, evaporate the filtrate to the sixth of its volume, and saturate it completely with diluted sulphuric acid.

The butyric acid separates and floats on the surface; it is decanted with a siphon; but as the liquid contains some butyric acid, it is distilled until the whole has passed over. By adding to the distillate some dissolved chloride of calcium, a new quantity of butyric acid is obtained. These two quantities of acid are saturated by carbonate of soda, decomposed by diluted sulphuric acid, dried over chloride of calcium, and distilled. Thus butyric acid, nearly pure, is obtained; the weight of which is about a third of the weight of the sugar used.

To prepare with this substance butyric ether, or oil of pineapple, mix equal parts of absolute alcohol and butyric acid; to the mixture add a small quantity of sulphuric acid. The best proportions are:—

Alcohol	1 pound.
Butyric acid . . .	1 "
Sulphuric acid . . .	4 drachms.

Heat the mixture for a few minutes, and soon the butyric ether forms a bed at the surface of the liquor. Add then an equal volume of water, decant the upper part, and distil the liquid, which furnishes a new quantity of ether. Stir the ether with a weak alkaline solution to separate the free acid.

The second method does not supply so pure a product, which is always mixed with capric, caproic, etc. ethers. The process is as follows: Saponify fresh butter by a solution of potash at 1.12; the soap thus obtained is dissolved in alcohol, and to the solution an excess of concentrated sulphuric acid is added. The whole is distilled. A mixture of ethers is thus obtained, in which the butyric predominates, and is purified as indicated above. The commercial oil of pineapple is generally prepared by dissolving one quart of butyric ether in eight or ten quarts of pure spirit.

In Austria they prepare a rum ether, which is the body to which rum owes its peculiar flavor. Take of black oxide of manganese and sulphuric acid each 12 pounds, alcohol 26 pounds, strong acetic acid 10 pounds; mix, and distil 12 pints.

Oil of Pear.

. This oil is obtained by dissolving in alcohol he acetic ether of the potato oil. Crude potato oil cannot be used to prepare this product—it must first be purified; for this purpose it is stirred with a diluted alkaline solution, then carefully distilled, collecting the portions passing between 212° and 233° C. The etherefication is conducted as follows: Take 1 part of purified potato oil, 1½ part of acetate of soda, and from 1 to 1½ part of sulphuric acid. The whole, well mixed, is kept at a gentle heat for a few hours. Water is then added to the liquor; acetic ether, which is insoluble, separates, and is collected; the balance of the liquor is distilled to separate what may remain in the solution. The product is carefully washed, first with a weak solution of carbonate of soda, then with pure water.

By mixing 15 parts by weight of this ether, 1½ part of acetic ether, and 100 to 120 parts of alcohol, an essence is obtained which gives to the substances with which it is mixed the perfume of the Bèrgamot pear.

Oil of Apples.

An alcoholic solution of valerianic ether, prepared from fusel oil, is designated by the name of oil of apples. Sometimes this product is simply prepared by distilling crude fusel oil mixed with sulphuric acid and bichromate of potash, but a small quantity of a very impure ether is thus obtained, mixed with a large quantity of amylic alcohol. To obtain an article of good quality, it is preferable to operate by the following rational method, consisting in isolating the valerianic acid, and etherefying it by a second operation.

To prepare valerianic acid, take 1 part of purified fusel oil; mix it little by little with 3 parts sulphuric acid; then add 2 parts of water. Heat at the same time in a tubulated retort a solution of 2¼ parts of bichromate of potash in 4½ of water. Introduce slowly and in small portions the first liquid, keeping up a gentle ebullition in the retort. The distilled liquor is saturated with carbonate of soda and evaporated to dryness, to obtain valerianate of soda. It is this salt which is directly used to produce the ether.

For this purpose take 1 part in weight of fusel oil, and mix it carefully with an equal quantity of sulphuric acid; add 1½ part of dry valerianate of soda; keep the liquor for some time at a gentle heat over a water bath, being careful not to raise the temperature too high. By adding water the ether separates, and is purified in the same manner as the products above mentioned.

When this ether is diluted with five or six times its volume of alcohol, a product is obtained which has the very agreeable odor of apples.

Oil of Apricot.

This is obtained by distilling 100 parts of alcohol, 10 of caseum of almonds, and 3 of dextrine.

Oil of Melon.

This is a mixture of ether of wine and of cocinic acid obtained from coco oil.

Oil of Quince.

It was believed, until recently, that the peeling of quinces contained œnanthylate of ethyloxide. New researches, however, have led to the supposition that the odorous principle of quinces is derived from the ether of pelargonic acid. Mr. Wagner, by his late researches on the action of nitric acid upon oil of rue, has discovered that besides the fatty acids discovered by Gerhardt, pelargonic acid is formed. This process may be advantageously employed for the preparation of crude pelargonate of ethyloxide, which, on account of its extremely agreeable odor, may be applied as a fruit essence. For the preparation of the liquid, which may be named essence of quince, oil of rue is treated with double the quantity of very dilute nitric acid, and the mixture heated until it begins to boil. After some time two layers are observed in the liquid; the upper is brownish, and the lower consists of the products of the oxidation of oil of rue and the excess of nitric acid. The lower layer is freed from the greater part of its nitric acid by evaporation in a bath of chloride of zinc. The white flocks frequently found in the acid liquid, which are probably fatty acids, are separated by filtration. The filtrate is mixed with spirits, and being digested at a gentle heat, by which a fluid is formed which has the agreeable odor of the quince in the highest degree, and may be purified by distillation.

Oil of Cucumber.

This may be obtained by distilling a solution of dextrine, and adding to the distillate a little ether of wine.

Oil of Hungary Wine.

This delicious aroma, which for a long time was kept secret, is nothing but a mixture of ether of wine with œnanthic acid.

Artificial Oil of Lemon.

Spirit of turpentine, treated in the following manner, forms a very curious hydrate:—

Spirit of turpentine . . .	1 gallon.
Rectified alcohol . . .	3 quarts.
Nitric acid	1 quart.

Agitate the mixture in a glass or earthen vessel, and let it rest. After one month the reaction is complete, and a large quantity of hydrate of spirit of turpentine is obtained. This hydrate, mixed with alcohol, produces voluminous crystals.

Submitted to the action of hydrochloric acid gas, the hydrate of turpentine loses a part of its water of crystallization and is transformed into a hydrochlorate having all the properties of the *camphor of lemon.* When heated it loses a part of its acid; then, treated by potassium, it is transformed into a fluid colorless oil, possessing the odor and chemical properties of natural lemon oil.

Essence of Mirbane.

This product, which is sometimes designated in the trade by the name of artificial oil of bitter almonds, does not belong to the series of ethers; it is a very different compound. The essence of mirbane, indeed, is due to the action of nitric acid on benzin, and is called by chemists *nitro-benzin.*

The first method followed in England to prepare it, was invented by Mansfield. His apparatus consists of a large glass tube, having the form of a worm; at its upper part it is divided into two branches, each one receiving a funnel. A stream of concentrated nitric acid runs slowly into one of the funnels; the other receives the benzin. The two liquids meet, and the reaction takes place with disengagement of heat. In following the worm the nitro-benzin cools; it is collected at the lower part, mixed with a certain quantity of nitric acid in excess.

Now, the operation is more simple; the attack of the benzin takes place in open vessels. Into large earthen jars or demijohns fuming nitric acid is introduced. The benzin, in proper quantity, is then poured on little by little, stirring all the time. The proportion of nitric acid varies according to the quality of the benzin, and cannot be exactly determined *à priori*, but experience teaches that the addition of benzin must be continued until the warm solution of nitro-benzin in nitric acid marks 24° to 25° by the acid hydrometer. At each addition of the benzin the reaction is energetic; the mass swells, and disengages large quantities of nitrous acid vapors; and the operator must be careful to wait until the ebullition has ceased before adding new material. Continue thus until all the benzin has been used. Allowed to cool, the nitro-benzin separates by degrees; to render the separation more complete, add to the liquid a quantity of water equal to five or six times its volume.

When the nitro-benzin is deposited, decant the upper liquid. To purify it, wash it at first with water, then with a weak solution of carbonate of soda, and a last time with water. For the use of the perfumer, this essence must be rectified. This operation is accomplished by passing through the product a current of steam, which carries with it all the nitro-benzin contained in the liquid.

To conclude all that is necessary to say in relation to the artificial essential oils, we shall present the reader with a table giving the proportions of the different substances used in making the essences of fruits. In this table each number represents, in volume, the quantity to be added to 100 parts in volume of alcohol.

Names of the essences.	Chloroform.	Nitric ether.	Aldehyde.	Acetate of ethyl.	Formate of ethyl.	Butyrate of ethyl.	Valerianate of ethyl.	Benzoate of ethyl.	Œnanthylate of ethyl.	Sebate of ethyl.	Salicylate of methyl.	Amylic alcohol.	Acetate of amyl.	Butyrate of amyl.	Valerianate of amyl.	Oil of lemon.	Oil of orange.	Alcohol solution saturated with				Glycerin.
																		Tartaric acid.	Oxalic acid.	Succinic acid.	Benzoic acid.	
Pineapple	1	...	1	...	...	5	...	...	...	...	...	...	...	10	...	...	...	...	...	...	...	3
Melon	...	...	2	...	1	4	5	...	...	10	...	...	...	...	...	...	...	...	...	...	...	3
Strawberry	...	1	...	5	1	5	...	...	...	...	1	...	3	2	...	...	...	...	...	...	...	2
Raspberry	...	1	1	5	1	1	...	1	1	1	1	...	1	1	...	...	...	5	...	1	...	4
Currant	...	...	1	5	...	...	...	1	1	...	...	...	...	...	...	...	...	5	...	1	1	...
Grape	2	...	2	...	2	...	...	...	10	...	1	...	...	...	...	...	...	5	...	3	...	10
Apple	1	1	2	1	...	...	...	...	...	...	...	...	...	...	10	...	...	...	1	...	...	4
Orange	2	...	2	5	1	1	...	1	...	...	1	...	10	...	...	...	10	1	...	...	...	10
Pear	...	...	...	5	...	...	...	...	...	...	...	...	10	...	...	...	...	...	...	...	...	10
Lemon	1	1	2	10	...	...	...	...	...	...	...	...	...	...	10	...	...	10	...	1	...	5
Black cherry	...	...	...	10	...	...	...	5	2	...	...	...	...	...	...	...	...	...	1	...	2	...
Cherry	...	...	...	5	...	...	...	5	1	...	...	...	...	...	...	...	...	...	...	...	1	3
Rum	...	...	5	5	1	2	...	...	4	...	...	...	...	...	...	...	...	...	...	...	...	8
Apricot	1	...	...	...	...	10	5	...	1	...	2	...	...	1	...	...	...	1	...	...	...	4
Peach	...	...	2	5	5	5	5	...	5	1	2	...	...	...	...	...	...	...	...	...	...	5

SECTION IV.

DISTILLED WATERS.

Distilled waters may be prepared from fresh or dried vegetables. In the latter case, only half the weight of the material should be used. They may also be prepared, for the most part, by agitating volatile oils with water, and filtering the solution; but waters obtained by this method have not so fine a flavor as those obtained from the distillation of the plants.

The distilled waters chiefly used are those prepared from aromatic plants, the volatile oils of which rise with the aqueous vapor and are condensed in the receiver; but as water is capable of holding but a small proportion of oil in solution, these preparations are generally feeble. In their preparation dry plants are sometimes used, but the fresh ones, especially of herbs or flowers, should be preferred. Flowers which lose their odor by desiccation may be preserved by incorporating them intimately with one-third of their weight of salt, and in this state afford distilled waters of a very delicate flavor. Certain practical rules have to be observed in conducting the process of distillation. When the substance employed is hard, dry, and fibrous, it should be mechanically divided and macerated in water for a short time previous to the operation. The quantity of material should not bear too large a proportion to the capacity of the alembic, as otherwise the water may boil over. The water should be brought quickly to the boiling point, and maintained in this state until the end of the operation. Care should be taken to leave sufficient water undistilled to cover the whole of the vegetable matter; but a portion of the latter should come in contact with the sides of the alembic above the water, and be thus exposed to igneous decomposition. To obviate this disadvantage the heat may be applied by means of an oil bath, regulated by a thermometer; or a bath of a solution of chloride of calcium, by which any temperature may be obtained between 212° and 270°; or, when the process is conducted upon a large scale, by means of steam introduced under pressure around the still.

But, however carefully the process may be conducted, the distilled waters prepared from plants always have at first an unpleasant smoky odor. They may be freed from this by exposure for a short time to the air before being inclosed in well-ground stopped bottles, in which they should be preserved. When long kept they are apt to become sour. The preventive of this decomposition is re-distillation. When thus purified they may be kept several years unchanged.

Another process is to impregnate the water with the volatile oil by trituration with carbonate of magnesia and filtration. This is by far the most simple and easy process. The resulting solution is pure and permanent, and is perfectly transparent. Chalk and sugar answer the same purpose, but the latter, by being dissolved with the oil, renders the preparation impure. In all cases the water used should be pure. Distilled waters are sometimes designated by the names of double, triple, quadruple; these names indicate the number of the distillations and the quality of the product.

CHAPTER IX.

FORMULÆ OF DISTILLED WATERS.

Rose Water.

THE *pale rose*, as the richest in perfume, is selected to make the water. It must be collected in the morning in dry weather. After having separated the leaves, they are introduced into an earthen jar, and one quart of water for every pound is poured upon them. Some add one ounce of salt, and allow it to macerate until the next day. The flowers are placed upon a diaphragm in a metallic cloth, or on a bed of straw spread on the bottom of the alembic. If six or eight pounds of roses are used, they must be covered with double their weight of water. This done, take the alembic, adapt the receiver, and heat slowly to 212°. The distillation then takes place. Be careful to keep the refrigeratory always cold.

To obtain a rose water of good quality, only half of the water poured into the alembic is distilled. Six quarts of water will give three quarts, etc. If more is distilled, the water will be less odoriferous.

The *durable* water is obtained by substituting fresh flowers for those which have already been submitted to distillation, the water of the first distillation being used instead of ordinary water. A new distillation is made, and the water thus obtained is very sweet.

The following waters may be obtained by the same process:—

Jonquil,	Lily of the Valley,
Nymphea.	Wild Poppy, etc.

Orange Flower Water.

Place in the cucurbit, as indicated above, two pounds of flower and nine pounds of distilled water. To obtain the double and treble water, operate as for rose water. It has been ascertained that orange flower water contains a little acetic acid. It is well to add to the water, before the distillation, a little powdered magnesia, so as to neutralize the acid. The following waters are obtained in the same manner:—

Wormwood,	Origanum,
Camomile.	Sweet Basil.

Lavender Water.

Fresh flowers of lavender . . 2 pounds.
Water . . . a sufficient quantity.

Distil until one quart is obtained.

Prepare in the same manner the waters of

Sage. Ground Ivy. Thyme, etc.

Anis Water.

Aniseed . . . . . . 2 pounds.
Water . . . . a sufficient quantity.

Distil so as to obtain one pint of product.

Prepare in the same manner the waters of

Parsely Seeds,	Badiane,
Fennel Seeds,	Juniper Berries,
Angelica Seeds.	Valerian Root.

Cinnamon Water.

Ceylon cinnamon . . 2 pounds.
Water . . . . a sufficient quantity.

Macerate twelve hours; distil afterwards at a gentle heat until four quarts are obtained.

Prepare in the same manner the waters of

Sassafras,	Cloves,
Cascarilla,	Pimento, etc.

Peppermint Water.

Fresh peppermint tops . 4 pounds.
Water . . . . . 12 "

Distil until two quarts are obtained. To render this water stronger, pour back the two quarts of water into the alembic, and distil anew until three pints are obtained.

Prepare in the same manner the water of

Hyssop,	Mint,
Marjoram,	Melissa, etc.

Cherry Laurel Water.

Fresh laurel leaves . .	4 pounds.
Water	8 "

Bruise the leaves before introducing them into the alembic, add the water, and distil until two quarts are obtained.

The leaves of peach, almond trees, and willow, are distilled in the same manner; as also the milky waters of orange, bergamot, aniseed, etc.

Bitter Almond Water.

Magma, or cake of bitter almonds	2 pounds.
Cold water	4 "

Dilute the almonds in water, so as to obtain a thin paste, which is introduced into the alembic. Allow it to macerate twenty-four hours, and distil until two quarts of water are obtained. When cold, filter to separate the undissolved oil.

Lemon Milky Water.

Fresh lemon zest . .	3 pounds.
Water	6 "
Alcohol	4 ounces.

Macerate two days and nights in the water and alcohol; then distil until three pints are obtained.

Bean-flower Water.

Fresh bean flowers . .	2 pounds.
Water	4 "

Macerate one night, and next day distil over a water bath.

Lily Water.

Fresh lily flowers . .	2 pounds.
Storax	2 ounces.
Water	6 pounds.

Macerate eight hours in water, and distil.

Anagallis Water.

Anagallis	4 pounds.
Benzoin	1 ounce.
Water	8 pounds.

Macerate twelve hours, and distil.

Lettuce Water.

Fresh lettuce . . .	10 pounds.
Water	20 "

Distil, at a gentle heat, until five quarts are obtained.

Prepare in the same manner the waters of

Plantain. Borage. Parietary, etc.

Cochlearia Water.

Fresh cochlearia leaves .	2 pounds.
Water . .	a sufficient quantity.

Distil at a gentle heat until one quart is obtained.

COLORED WATERS FOR SHOP WINDOWS.

White Water.

Water	2 pints.
Amygdaline soap . . .	3 drachms.
Cucumber pomade . .	3 ounces.

Mix the soap with the pomade, and add to the water little by little.

Fine Blue Water.—Solution of sulphate of copper in water, to which has been added an excess of ammonia.

Prussian Blue Water.

Prussian blue . . .	8 grains.
Oxalic acid . . .	16 "
Water	16 ounces.

Yellow Water.—Acid solution of chromate of potash with some carbonate of potash.

Lilac Water.—Add a solution of carbonate of ammonia to a solution of nitrate of cobalt until the precipitate is dissolved. Add a little of ammoniacal sulphate of copper.

Purple Water.

Sulphate of copper . .	1 ounce.
Carbonate of ammonia . .	1½ "
Water	2 pounds.

Red Water.—Solution of bichromate of potash.

Another.—Carmine, dissolved in ammonia; decoction of madder, with a little carbonate of ammonia; infusion of wild poppy flowers.

Violet Water.—Mixture of ammonia and sulphate of copper and lilac water.

Green Water.—Mixture of sulphate of copper and hydrochloric acid.

Others. — Solution of sulphate of copper, to which is added hypochlorite of soda; solution of a salt of nickel; mixture of sulphate of copper and bichromate of potash.

SECTION V.

ALCOHOLATES, OR SPIRITS.—TINCTURES.

ALCOHOL dissolves many odoriferous principles and keeps them well, especially the odors extracted from resinous substances. But it does not dissolve well the odoriferous principles of flowers belonging to certain families, such as lilacs, acacia, etc. Hence the reason for fatty bodies being used to extract and fix their perfume. The alcoholates, designated by perfumers under the name of *spirits,* are obtained by macerating for a few days the aromatic substances in rectified spirits, and distilling them afterwards over a water-bath. Substances such as fruits, seeds, and barks, ought to be coarsely ground before maceration. The alcohol used must be stronger when the plant contains a large amount of water of vegetation. The distillation is done over a water bath until three-quarters of the alcohol used has passed over. The alcoholates of roses may be entirely distilled.

CHAPTER X.

SPIRITS.

Spirit of Mint.

Fresh tops and leaves of mint	2 pounds.
Alcohol at 95°	3 quarts.
Distilled water of mint . .	1 quart.

Macerate four or five days, distil over a water bath until two and a half quarts are obtained.

Marjoram Spirit.

Fresh leaves of marjoram . .	2 pounds.
Alcohol at 95°	3 quarts.
Distilled water of marjoram .	1 quart.

Macerate five days; pour into an alembic and distil two and a half quarts.

Prepare in the same manner the alcoholates of sweet basil, hyssop, lavender, wormwood, melisse, thyme.

Spirit of Rhodium.

Rhodium wood . . .	2 pounds.
Alcohol at 95°	4 quarts.

Macerate twenty-five days, stirring several times a day. Decant and distil three quarts over a water bath.

Another.

Oil of rhodium wood .	2 ounces.
Rectified alcohol . .	2 quarts.

Pour the oil into the alcohol, digest three days, stirring from time to time. Filter and keep in well-corked bottles.

Spirit of Cloves.

Cloves	8 ounces.
Alcohol	2 quarts.

Macerate fifteen days and filter. If instead of filtering it is distilled, the spirit obtained will be sweeter.

The same process may be used to procure the spirits of

Badiane or Staranise,
Anise,
Ambrette,
Cinnamon,
Sandal, etc.

Spirit of Lemon.

Fresh lemon peel . .	1 pound.
Alcohol at 90° . . .	3 quarts.

Macerate ten days, and distil to dryness.

Prepare in the same manner the alcoholates of bergamot, orange, cedrat, etc.

Alcoholate or Spirituous Water of Roses.

Fresh roses . . .	2 pounds.
Alcohol at 95° . . .	2 quarts.
Water	1 pint.

Macerate the flowers one night, next day distil over a water bath. If a stronger spirituous water is wanted, redistil the product of the first distillation with two pounds of fresh roses.

Spirituous Water of Orange Flowers.

Fresh orange flowers . .	2 pounds.
Alcohol at 95° . . .	3 pints.
Water	1 pint.

Macerate twelve hours, and distil over a water bath. By redistilling the product obtained from the first distillation with one pound of fresh flowers, the water is double.

Spirit of Castor.

Castor	1 ounce.
Alcohol	3 pints.

Macerate a few days, and distil over a water bath.

Aromatic Ammoniacal Alcoholate.

Cinnamon	2½ drachms.
Cloves	4 "
Lemon peel	4 ounces.
Carbonate of potash .	8 "
Sal ammoniac . . .	4 "
Alcohol	2 quarts.

Macerate six days in alcohol, then add two quarts of water; distil over a water bath until three quarts are obtained.

Compound Alcoholate of Honey.

White honey . . .	11 ounces.
Cloves	1 ounce.
Nutmegs	6 drachms.
Coriander . . .	10 ounces.
Cardamom . . .	1 ounce.
Benzoin	6 drachms.
Storax	6 "
Tolu	6 "
Vanilla	5 "
Lemon zest . . .	2 ounces.
Alcohol at 95° . .	2 quarts.

Macerate the whole, except the honey, for five days. Express, and to the product add

Rose water . . .	8 ounces.
Orange-flower water . .	8 "

then add the honey; stir well, and distil over a water bath.

CHAPTER XI.

AROMATIC TINCTURES.

THESE tinctures consist of alcohol, holding in solution one or more aromatic principles.

Tincture of Benzoin.

Coarsely-powdered benzoin	8 ounces.
Alcohol at 95°	2½ quarts.

Macerate until all the benzoin is dissolved, stirring several times a day. Filter, and keep in well-closed bottles.

Tincture of Balsam of Peru.

Liquid balsam of Peru .	8 ounces.
Alcohol at 95°	3 pints.

Macerate, and, when completely dissolved, filter.

Tincture of Balsam of Tolu.

Balsam of Tolu	5 ounces.
Alcohol	3 pints.

Filter after complete solution.

Tincture of Storax.

Storax	5 ounces.
Alcohol at 95°	3 pints.

Filter after the solution is complete.

Tincture of Liquidamber.

Liquidamber	. . .	5 ounces.
Alcohol at 60°	. . .	3 pints.

Dissolve and filter.

These resinous solutions are of great importance in perfumery in the manufacture of many scented compounds, waters, pomades, and perfumes. In the same manner, tinctures of myrrh, guaiacum, galbanum, mastic, etc. are prepared. Some balsams, such as those of Mecca, Chio, and Canada, are but little soluble in pure alcohol, but are dissolved in diluted alcohol.

Tincture of Grain of Paradise.

Coarsely-powdered grain	.	4 ounces.
Alcohol at 95°	. . .	1 pint.

Macerate fifteen days, pass through a cloth, press, and filter.

The following tinctures are prepared in the same manner:—

Cardamom,	Coriander,	Galanga,
Nutmegs,	Pyrethrum,	Ginger.
Mace, etc.		

Tincture of Vanilla.

Vanilla	. . . .	4 ounces.
Alcohol	. . . .	1 quart.

Cut the vanilla in small pieces, and macerate it

for thirty or forty days, being careful to stir every day; after this time filter. It may be obtained colorless by distilling over a water bath.

Tincture of Musk.

Musk	1 ounce.
Alcohol at 36°	1 pint.

Introduce into a warm mortar the musk, with half an ounce of sugar. Powder carefully; add the alcohol little by little so as to divide well. When the tincture is homogeneous, pour it into a bottle and macerate two weeks. Filter.

Another.

Musk	1 ounce.
Tincture of ambergris .	2 ounces.
" vanilla . .	2 "
Alcohol	14 "

Rub the musk as above; add the tinctures and alcohol; macerate one month; filter two or three times, and to the product add a few drops of oil of roses.

This tincture is superior to the above.

Tinctures of Civet and Castor are prepared as the tincture of musk. To render them more agreeable, add a little ambergris and vanilla.

Tincture of Ambergris.

Ambergris	. . .	1 ounce.
Sugar	. . . .	½ "

Rub together in a mortar as we have said for the musk; add—

Tincture of civet or musk	.	3½ ounces.
Alcoholate of roses	. .	14 "

In which

Carbonate of potash	. .	½ ounce,

has been dissolved. Macerate one month, and filter.

CHAPTER XII.

COMPOUND TINCTURES.

Aromatic Tincture; called The Three Aromatics.

Coarsely-powdered nutmegs	2 ounces.
" " cloves .	2 "
" " cinnamon	1½ ounce.
Flowers of pomegranate .	1½ "
Alcohol	1 quart.

Macerate ten days, and filter.

Tincture of Arnica.

Coarsely-powdered flowers of arnica	2 ounces.
Coarsely-powdered cloves .	5 drachms.
" " cinnamon	4 "
" " anis . .	4 "
Alcohol	1 quart.

Macerate ten days. Filter.

Aromatic Tincture, called Cephalic.

Coarsely-powdered nutmegs	.	2 ounces.
" " cloves	.	2 "
" " ginger	.	2 "
" " pepper	.	2 "
Cinnamon . .	.	½ ounce.
Alcohol	.	1 quart.

Macerate ten days, and filter. Add—

Acetic acid . .	.	½ ounce.

Laurel Tincture.

Laurel leaves . . .	.	4 ounces.
Cloves	.	½ ounce.
Pepper	.	½ "
Alcoholate of lavender	.	4 ounces.
" parsley	.	4 "

Macerate ten days in the two alcoholates; filter. Used in lotions for the hands.

Aromatic Ethereal Tincture.

Coarsely-powdered cinnamon	2½ drachms.
" " ginger .	1¼ drachm.
" " nutmegs	1¼ "
" " pepper .	1¼ "
" " cardamom	2½ drachms.
Ether	16 ounces.

Macerate six days. Filter.

Use as a remedy in fainting fits.

Prepare in the same manner the ethereal tinctures which contain musk, ambergris, castoreum, civet, and the different balsams.

Polyaromatic Tincture, or Hoffmann's Balsam of Life.

Oil of cinnamon,
" lemon,
" cloves,
" lavander,
" mace,
" marjoram,
" neroli, each . . ¾ drachm.
Tinct. of musk amber . . ½ "
Alcohol . . . . . 16 ounces.

Macerate ten hours. Filter.

Another for Contusions.

Fresh leaves of sweet basil,
" hyssop,
" marjoram,
" melisse,
" mint,
" origanum,
" rosemary,
" sage,
" thyme,
" wormwood,
" angelica,

Fresh leaves of rue,
" fennel,
Tops of hypericum,
" lavender, each . . 1 ounce.
Alcohol at 95° . . . 3 pints.

Macerate ten days and filter. If this tincture is distilled, and to the distillate a little tincture of musk is added, a very sweet scented water is obtained.

SECTION VI.

ALCOHOLIC EXTRACTS OF FLOWERS WITH FUGITIVE ODORS.

FLOWERS with fugitive odors give only by distillation a very feeble product. Thus, when water or alcohol is distilled from lilies, tuberose, narcissus, jonquil, or violets, a very weak perfume is obtained which evaporates in a very short time. Fixed oils and fatty bodies being the better excipients for these delicate perfumes, are employed to fix them, and afterwards pure alcohol is used to extract them from these fatty substances.*

* The principal seat of manufacture is in the South of France, at Grasse and Cannes, where it is conducted on a very large scale. The oils and greases, after being impregnated with the perfume of flowers, are sold to the perfumers, who prepare from them pomades and extracts.

CHAPTER XIII.

PROCESSES FOR THE MANUFACTURE OF EXTRACTS.

THERE are two processes for the manufacture of extracts. The first consists in macerating flowers in fresh oils or greases for ten or fifteen days, then to treat these oils or greases by a certain quantity of alcohol at 95°. The mixture is allowed to macerate for fifteen days, being careful to stir several times a day. After this time decant the oil which floats on the surface, and when the separation is effected filter the alcohol through paper to deprive it of all oily particles. These operations must always be performed in glass or porcelain jars.

Second Process.—When the greases or fixed oils have deprived the flowers of their perfume they are digested in alcohol as above, and the perfumed spirit is drawn off by distilling. In this manner the extracts are entirely deprived of that fatty taste which is found in poor extracts.

Process by Impregnation, called Enfleurage.

This process requires a box lined with galvanized sheet iron, frames, and woollen or cotton cloths which are to be fixed on the frames. The apparatus must be very clean. The whole being ready, begin by dipping the cloth in fresh olive, behn or almond oil, press out the excess of oil, and fix the cloth on the frame, spread a bed of flowers over it, then slide the frame in the box, dip a second cloth in the oil and operate as for the first. Continue thus until the box is entirely filled with frames. Close the box in such a manner that the top will gently press on the flowers. Allow it to stand twenty-four hours. After this time the flowers are thrown away and substituted by fresh ones, operating in the same manner as before. It is necessary to repeat the operation five or six times, and even more with some delicate flowers, until the oil is entirely saturated with the essential oil. The cloths are then steeped in rectified alcohol and subjected to the action of the press to extract all the oil. This done, pour the mixed oil and alcohol into an alembic, stir well and distil over a water bath. Soon the alcohol, saturated with the essential oil, begins to distil over, and the fixed oil is left in the alembic. Such is the process of preparing the scented alcoholates known in perfumery under the name of *extracts*.

The following are obtained by this process:—

Cassia,	Lilac,	Syringa,
Jasmine,	Lily,	Tuberose,
Hyacinth,	Pink,	Violet, etc. etc.
Jonquil,	Reseda,	

If instead of washing the woollen cloths in alcohol, they are pressed and the oil collected, perfumed oils, such as are manufactured in Provence and Italy, are obtained.

Oils thus perfumed used to be the fashion, but now greases are preferred. These extracts may also be obtained by the following process without distillation:—

In a glass bottle mix equal parts of scented oil and alcohol at 95°, that is, 1 lb. of oil and 1 lb. of alcohol. Shake the bottle briskly so as to render the liquid milky; then place the bottle in ice, or, if in winter, expose it to the frost. The oil solidifies, the alcohol saturated with essential oil separates and occupies the upper part of the bottle. The alcohol is decanted, and an extract obtained.

SECTION VII.

MIXTURES OF EXTRACTS AND AROMATIC TINCTURES TO OBTAIN SCENTED WATERS.

THE harmonious combination of perfumed oils, tinctures, aromatic spirits, and other odoriferous compounds, produces an immense variety of scented waters, more or less sweet, of which we shall give the principal formulæ.

CHAPTER XIV.

FORMULÆ FOR SCENTED WATERS.

Eau de Jasmin.

Alcohol at 90°	2 quarts.
Extract of jasmine . .	1 quart.
Tincture of Tolu . .	4 drachms.
" benzoin . .	4 "
" ambergris . . .	1¼ drachm.

Agitate briskly, permit it to stand one night, and filter.

Eau de Reseda.

Alcohol at 90° . . .	2 quarts.
Extract of reseda . .	1 quart.
" rose . . .	1 ounce.
Tincture of ambergris .	2 drachms.
" Tolu . .	4 "

Shake well, let it stand twenty-four hours, and filter.

Eau de Tubereuse.

Alcohol	2 quarts.
Extract of tuberose . .	1 quart.
Spirituous water of rose .	1 pint.
Tincture of Tolu . .	4 drachms.
" ambergris .	1¼ drachm.

Shake thoroughly, and after twelve hours filter.

Eau de Violettes.

Alcohol at 90° . . .	2 quarts.
Extract of violet . .	1 quart.
" cassia . .	1 pint.
Spirituous water of roses .	1 "
Tincture of ambergris .	1¼ drachm.

Operate as above.

Eau de Jacinthe.

Alcohol	2 quarts.
Extract of jacinth . .	1 quart.
Spirituous water of orange flower	1 pint.
Tincture of benzoin . .	1¼ drachm.
" ambergris .	1¼ "

Operate as above.

Eau de Jonquille.

Alcohol	2 quarts.
Extract of jonquille . .	1 quart.
Spirituous water of orange flower	1 pint.
Spirituous water of reseda .	1 "
Tincture of ambergris .	1¼ drachm.

Operate as above.

Prepare in the same manner all scented wate of fugitive odoriferous flowers.

Eau d'Héliotrope.

Spirituous water of rose .	1 pound.
" " jasmine .	1 "
" " tuberose	1 "
Tincture of vanilla . .	8 ounces.
" balsam of Peru	4 "
" ambergris . .	1 ounce.

Allow it to stand a few hours, and filter.

Eau de Vanille.

Tincture of vanilla . .	1 quart.
" balsam of Tolu	8 ounces.
" ambergris and musk . .	2 "
Rose water	8 "

Mix and filter.

Eau de Myrte.

Oil of myrtle . . .	2 ounces.
Alcohol	24 "
Distilled water of flowers and leaves of myrtle . .	8 "
Orange-flower water . .	4 "
Rose water	4 "

Stir and filter.

*Extrait de Fleurs de Peches.**

Alcohol	1 quart.
Spirituous water of orange flower	1 pint.
Oil of bitter almonds . .	1 drachm.
" lemon . . .	1 "
Tincture of balsam of Peru	2½ drachms.

Let it stand a few hours, and filter.

* Extract of Peach Blossoms.

SECTION VIII.

COMPOUND PERFUMES AND COSMETICS MOST EMPLOYED.

CHAPTER XV.

PERFUMED ALCOHOLATES.

Eau de Cologne (*Supérieure*).

Oil of lemon	. . .	12½ drachms.
" cedrat	. . .	2½ "
" bergamot	. . .	2½ "
" lavender	. . .	5 "
" Portugal	. . .	2 "
" rosemary	. . .	1¼ drachm.
" white thyme	. .	1¼ "
" mint	. . .	2½ drachms.
" vervain	. . .	1¼ drachm.
" small orange	. .	1¼ "
Alcohol at 95°	. . .	3 pints.
Alcoholate of melissa	. .	1 pound.
Tincture of ambretta	. .	8 ounces.

Shake the bottle well, so as to effect the solution of the oils. Let it rest six hours, then add—

Tincture of ambergris	.	2½ drachms.

Filter several times, until a clear liquid is obtained. By distilling this mixture, the preparation will be finer and sweeter.

Another (*Treble*).

Oil of cedrat . . .	4½ drachms.
" bergamot . . .	3 "
" lemon . . .	3 "
" neroli . . .	1 drachm.
" Portugal . . .	2 drachms.
" vervain . . .	1 drachm.
" mint	1¼ "
" rosemary . . .	1 "
" thyme . . .	1 "
Alcohol at 95° . . .	1 pint.
Alcoholate of melissa . .	1 "
Tincture of musk . .	12 drops.

Shake the mixture, let it rest twelve hours, and filter until clear.

Another (Codex).

Oil of bergamot	. . .	2 ounces.
" lemon	. . .	3 "
" orange	. . .	1 ounce.
" neroli	. . .	1 "
" cedrat	. . .	1 "
" rosemary	. . .	1 "
" lavender	. . .	½ "
" orange flower	. .	½ "
" cinnamon	. .	3 drachms.
Spirit of rosemary	. .	8 ounces.
Compound water melisse	.	3 pounds.
Alcohol at 95°	. . .	12 "

Distil over a water bath until nearly dry, and add—

Eau de bouquet	. . .	1 pound.

Another.

Oil of Portugal	. . .	1½ ounce.
" bergamot	. . .	1½ "
" cedrat	. . .	1 "
" lemon	. . .	1 "
" neroli	. . .	1½ "
" " petit grain	.	1 "
" rosemary	. . .	2 ounces.
" lavender	. . .	2 "
" benzoin	. . .	2 "

Infuse the whole for two weeks in rectified alcohol, stirring the mixture three or four times a day. Distil twice. The product will be one quart of fine concentrated Cologne water.

Another (*Plenet*).

Alcohol at 90° . . .	24	pounds.
Oil of neroli . . .	16	grains.
" lemon . . .	7	"
" bergamot . . .	7	"
" cedrat . . .	7	"
Water de la Reine de Hongrie	7	"
" lavender . . .	2	"
" vulnerary . . .	3	"
" rosemary . . .	2	"

Another (*cheap*).

Mix three quarts of alcohol at 95° with one drachm each of the following oils:—

Rosemary,	Cedrat,	Lemon.
Bergamot,	Neroli,	

Filter, and keep for use.

Eau de Lavande (*English*).

Oil of lavender . . .	3	drachms.
" bergamot . . .	3	"
" roses . . .	6	drops.
" cloves . . .	6	"
" rosemary . . .	$\frac{3}{4}$	drachm.
Tincture of musk . .	$\frac{3}{4}$	"
Benzoic acid . . .	$\frac{1}{2}$	"
Honey	1	ounce.
Alcohol	1	pint.
Spirituous water of rose .	2	ounces.

Stir well; let it rest six hours; filter.

Another.

Rectified alcohol . . .	25 ounces.
Rose water . . .	12½ "
Oil of bergamot . . .	1 drachm.
Ambergris . . .	3 grains.
Aqua ammonia . . .	½ drachm.
Musk	3 grains.
Oil of lavender . . .	4 drachms.
Flowers " . . .	1 ounce.

Distil so as to obtain one quart of product.

Eau de Lavande Ambrée.

Lavender flowers . .	3 pounds.
Fresh lemon peel . .	5 ounces.
Rhodium wood . . .	2 "
Alcohol	3 pounds.

Digest eight days, and distil over a water bath.

Introduce the distillate in a large bottle, and add—

Alcoholate of roses.
Spirit of thyme.
" rosemary.
Tincture of musk amber.
Distillate of water of roses.

Let it stand twenty-four hours; filter several times until perfectly clear.

Eau de Bouquet.

Odoriferous alcohol from honey	2 ounces.
Alcoholate of jasmine . .	5 drachms.
" cloves . .	4 "
" violet . .	4 "
" calamus aromaticus	2 "
" lavender . .	2 "
" orange flower .	½ drachm.

Mix; stir well; allow it to rest a few days; filter.

Another.

Oil of cloves . . .	½ drachm.
Tincture of cloves . .	2 drachms.
Oil of bergamot . . .	2 "
" thyme . . .	¼ drachm.
Alcohol at 95° . . .	1 quart.

Dissolve, stir, and add—

Extract of jasmine . .	8 ounces.
" rose . . .	4 "
" jonquil . .	4 "
" violet . .	4 "
" tuberose . .	4 "
" reseda . .	4 "
" orange flower .	4 "
" cassia . .	4 "

Stir the mixture well; then add—

Tincture of musk amber .	2 drachms.
" vanilla benzoin	2 "

Digest five hours, and filter.

Eau de Mille Fleurs.

Oil of neroli . . .	½ drachm.
" cloves . . .	1 "
Tincture of vanilla . .	1 ounce.
Alcohol	1 quart.

Stir, to dissolve the oils. Then add—

Eau de bouquet . . .	1 quart.
" roses . . .	1 pint.
" fleur d'oranger .	8 ounces.
Tincture of ambergris and musk	1 drachm.

Stir anew, and, after a few hours' rest, filter.

Eau des Odalisques.

Oil of lemon . . .	4 drachms.
" bergamot . . .	2½ "
" cedrat . . .	2½ "
Tincture of ambergris and musk	1¼ drachm.
Vervain water . . .	8 ounces.
Alcohol at 90° . . .	1 quart.

Another (*Bacheville*).

To prepare five quarts, take of—

Alcohol at 90° . . .	4 quarts.
Rose water . . .	1 quart.
Cochineal	½ drachm.
Cream tartar . . .	4 ounces.

Styrax	1½ ounce.
Liquid balsam of Peru .	5 drachms.
Dry " " . .	5 "
Galanga	1 ounce.
Pyrethrum root . . .	1½ "
Cyperus root . . .	1½ "
Vanilla	1 drachm.
Dry orange peel . . .	2 drachms.
Cinnamon	1 drachm.
Oil of mint . . .	1 "
Angelica root . . .	1 "
Anethum seeds . . .	1 "

Infuse eight days, and filter.

Eau des Bayaderes (*Naquet*).

Oil of bergamot . . .	4 ounces.
" lemon . . .	2 "
" Portugal . . .	2 "
" neroli . . .	1 ounce.
" " petit grain .	1 "
Powdered balsam of Tolu .	1 "
Oil of rosemary . . .	4 drachms.
" rose	20 drops.
Cochineal	4 drachms.

Infuse the whole for ten days in twelve quarts of alcohol at 95°, filter, and keep for use.

Eau de Chypre.

Mix—

Jasmine water . . .	1 quart.
Bergamot " . . .	1 "
Violet " . . .	1 "
Tuberose " . . .	1 "
Spirit of ambrette . .	1 pint.
Judea balsam . . .	1 ounce.
Storax	4 drachms.
Essence of musk . .	1 ounce.

Pour into the mixture two ounces of rose water, stir well, and filter.

Eau de la Reine de Hongrie.

In one quart of alcohol infuse—

Tops of rosemary . .	14 ounces.
" lavender . .	3½ "
" marjoram . .	3½ "

After a few days, express and filter.

Eau de Musc des Indes.

Mix—

Rectified alcohol . .	2 quarts.
Spirit of ambrette . .	1 quart.
Balsam of Tolu . . .	2 ounces.
Tincture of vanilla . .	1 ounce.
Essence of musk . .	1 "
" ambergris . .	2 drachms.

Rose water in sufficient quantity to render this perfume sweeter.

Incisif Parfumê (for the Nerves).

Compound alcoholate of melisse	. . . .	2¾ ounces.
Alcoholate of	cloves . .	1½ ounce.
"	lavender .	5 drachms.
"	cyperus .	5 "
"	sans pareil .	3½ ounces.
"	jasmin .	1½ ounce.
"	orris . .	1½ "
"	orange flower	6 drachms.

Mix, infuse a few hours, and filter.

Spirituous Water of Jasmine.

Introduce into a bottle—

Oil of jasmine . . .	8 ounces.
Rectified alcohol . . .	8 "

Let it infuse four days, stirring several times a day. Expose the bottle to artificial cold; the fixed oil solidifies, and precipitates to the bottom of the bottle. Decant the alcohol, which has taken all tho perfume contained in the oil.

Alcoholate of Orris.

Powdered orris . . .	4 ounces.
Rectified alcohol . .	16 "

Macerate two weeks, stirring often; filter. With the filtrate begin the same operation, that is, pour it on a fresh quantity of orris; macerate two weeks, and filter.

Extrait de Miel de Naples.

White honey . . .	4 pounds.
Pale roses	2 "
Orange flowers . . .	2 "

Rub the flowers with the honey, to form a paste, which is diluted with—

Rose water	3 quarts.

Let it ferment. When the acid fermentation begins, check it by pouring into it—

Alcoholate of rosemary .	1 quart.

Then add—

Mace	4 ounces.
Cloves	1 ounce.
Calamus aromaticus . .	2 ounces.
Storax	8 "
Benzoin	8 "
Orange and lemon peel .	8 "
Alcohol at 90° . . .	2 quarts.
Alcoholate of peach flower .	1 quart.
Distilled water of almonds .	1 pound.

Macerate eight days; pour the whole into the alembic, and distil.

To the distillate add—

Tincture of ambergris .	1 ounce.
" " musk . .	½ "

Eau de Miel Odorante (for Handkerchiefs).

White honey . . .	1 pound.
Coriander . . .	1 "
Fresh zest of lemon . .	1 ounce.
Cloves	6 drachms.
Nutmegs	1 ounce.
Benzoin	1 "
Storax	1 "
Rose water . . .	4 ounces.
Orange-flower water .	4 "
Alcohol at 95° . . .	3 pints.

Mix; infuse four days; pass through filter.

Eau de Miel Odorante de Londres.

Water	1 quart.
Honey	1 ounce.
Oil of bergamot . .	½ drachm.
" neroli . . .	¼ "
Tincture of ambergris .	¼ "
" saffron . .	8 ounces.

Eau des Sultanes.

Tincture of Balsam of Tolu .	4 ounces.
" " Peru .	4 "
" " benzoin .	4 "
" " styrax .	4 "
" " vanilla .	4 "
Rectified alcohol . . .	2 quarts.

Agitate to effect the solution of the mixture, then add—

Tincture of ambergris and musk	6 drachms.
Jonquil spirituous water . .	1 quart.
Hyacinth " " . .	1 "
Reseda " " . .	1 "

Infuse twenty-four hours, and filter.

Eau Sans Pareille.

Oil of lemon . . .	4 drachms.
" cedrat . . .	2 "
" bergamot . .	2½ "
Spirit of rosemary . .	8 ounces.
Tincture of ambergris .	2 drachms.
Rectified alcohol . .	2 quarts.

Distil over a water bath.

Eau de Toilette.

Alcohol at 70° . . .	28 ounces.
Benzoin	2½ drachms.
Incense	2½ "
Gum arabic . . .	2½ "
Cloves	1¼ drachm.
Nutmegs	1¼ "
Sweet almonds . . .	4 drachms.
Orris	4 "
Oil of rose	10 drops.
" bergamot . . .	10 "
" lemon . . .	10 "

Infuse twelve days; decant; pass through a cloth, and press; then filter.

Eau Impériale.

Infuse in four quarts of rectified alcohol—

Fresh violet flowers . .	4 ounces.
" hyacinth " . .	4 "
" jonquil " . .	4 "
Musk roses . . .	4 "
Tuberoses	2 "
Powdered orris . . .	2 "
" nutmegs . .	1 ounce.
" cloves . .	1 "
" sandal . .	2 ounces.

After a maceration of eight days, add—

Oil of Portugal . . .	4 drachms.
" bergamot . .	4 "
" lemon . . .	4 "
Tincture of ambergris and musk	2 "

Distil over a water bath until three quarts have passed over. The balance is preserved for perfumes of a second quality.

To these three quarts, add—

Jasmine water . . .	4 ounces.
Orange-flower water . .	4 "

Keep in well-corked bottles.

This perfume is one of the sweetest manufactured.

Essence Royale.

Ambergris	2.5 parts.
Musk	1.2 "
Civet	0.5 "
Oil of rose	0.2 "
" cinnamon . .	0.2 "
" rhodium . . .	0.2 "
" orange flower . .	0.3 "
Carbonate of potash . .	0.6 "
Alcohol at 90° . . .	86.0 "

Mix, stir, and filter. It is a perfume for the handkerchief.

Eau de la Duchesse.

Coarsely-powdered cinnamon .	1 ounce.
" " cloves .	1 "
" " sandal .	1 "
Benzoin	5 drachms.
Ambrette	5 "

Macerate for fifteen days in two quarts of alcohol at 90°, being careful to stir every day. Pass through a cloth, and to the filtrate add—

Spirit of pink . . .	4 ounces.
" violet . . .	4 "
" bergamot . .	4 "
" jasmine . .	4 "
" roses . . .	4 "

Tinct. of ambergris and musk, 2 drachms.

Filter several times until clear.

Eau Ambrée.

Alcohol	1 quart.
Spirit of ambrette . .	1 "
Tincture of ambergris . .	1 ounce.
" musk . .	4 drachms.
Orange-flower water . .	8 ounces.

Let it macerate a few hours; filter.

Eau d'Héliotrope Composée.

Tincture of vanilla . .	1 pound.
" balsam Peru .	8 ounces.
Spirit of roses . . .	1 pound.
" jasmine . . .	1 "
" tuberose . .	8 ounces.
" orange flowers .	8 "
Ess. of ambergris and musk,	2 drachms.

Stir, macerate a few hours, and filter.

Eau à la Frangipanne.

Alcohol . . .	2 quarts.
Extract of jasmine . .	1 quart.
Spirituous water of roses .	4 ounces.
Spirit of cassia . . .	4 "
Oil of bergamot . . .	2 "
" vanilla . . .	2 "
Tincture of Tolu . . .	1 ounce.
" Peru . . .	1 "
" saffron . .	2 ounces.
" ambergris and musk,	2 drachms.

Infuse five hours, stirring often. Filter.

Eau d'Aspasie.

Extract of jasmine	8	ounces.
" jonquil	8	"
" orange flowers	8	"
" violet	8	"
" tuberose	8	"
Tincture of balsam of Peru	4	drachms.
" balsam of Tolu	4	"
" ambergris and musk,	4	"

Mix, let it rest a few hours, and filter.

Eau de Laïs.

Eau de cologne	4	ounces.
" jasmin	2	"
" tuberose	2	"
" nard	2	"
" cyperus	2	"
" melisse	2	"
" lemon	2	"
Tincture of benzoin	1	ounce.
" vanilla	1	"
" musk amber	4	drachms.

Shake in a bottle, leave it to rest a few hours, and filter.

CHAPTER XVI.

BOUQUETS AND NOSEGAYS.

THESE compounds are mixtures of simple ottos in spirits, which, when properly blended, produce an agreeable and characteristic odor.

Alhambra Parfumê.

Extract of tuberose	. .	16 ounces.
" geranium	. .	8 "
" acacia	. .	4 "
" fleur d'orange	.	4 "
" civet	. .	4 "

Mix and filter.

Bosphorus Bouquet.

Extract of acacia	. .	16 ounces.
" jasmine	. .	8 "
" rose, triple	.	8 "
" fleur d'orange	.	8 "
" tuberose	. .	8 "
" civet	. .	4 "
Otto of almonds	. .	10 drops.

Mix and filter.

Bouquet d'Amour.

Esprit de rose (from pomade)	16 ounces.
" jasmin "	16 "
" violette "	16 "
" cassie "	16 "
Extract of musk . .	8 "
" ambergris .	8 "

Mix and filter.

Bouquet des Fleurs du Val d'Andorre.

Ext. de jasmin (from pomade)	16 ounces.
" rose "	16 "
" violette "	16 "
" tubereuse "	16 "
Extract of orris . . .	16 "
Oil of geranium . . .	2 drachms.

Mix and filter.

Buckingham Palace Bouquet.

Extrait de fleur d'orange, " " cassie, " " jasmin, " " rose,	from pomade, of each 16 ounces.
Extract of orris . . .	8 ounces.
" ambergris . .	8 "
Oil of neroli	30 drops.
" lavender . . .	30 "
" rose	1 drachm.

Mix and filter.

Bouquet des Delices.

Extrait de rose " violette " tubereuse	from pomade, of each 16 ounces.
Extract of orris . . .	8 ounces.
" ambergris . .	8 "
Oil of bergamot . . .	2 drachms.
Lemon zest . . .	4 "

Mix and filter.

Court Nosegay.

Extrait de rose . . .	16 ounces.
" violette . .	16 "
" jasmin . .	16 "
Esprit de rose, triple . .	16 "
Extract of musk . .	1 ounce.
" ambergris . .	1 "
Oil of lemon zest . .	4 drachms.
" bergamot . . .	4 "
" neroli . . .	1 drachm.

Mix and filter.

Empress Eugenie's Nosegay.

Extract of musk . .	4 ounces.
" vanilla . .	4 "
" tonquin bean .	4 "
" neroli . .	4 "
" geranium . .	8 "
" rose, triple .	8 "
" sandal . .	8 "

Mix and filter.

Esterhazy Bouquet.

Extrait de fleur d'orange (from pomade)	16	ounces.
Esprit de rose, triple	16	"
Extract of vitivert	16	"
" vanilla	16	"
" orris	16	"
" tonquin	16	"
Esprit de neroli	16	"
Extract of ambergris	8	"
Oil of sandal	30	drops.
" cloves	30	"

Mix and filter.

Ess. Bouquet.

Esprit de rose, triple	16	ounces.
Extract of ambergris	2	"
" orris	8	"
Oil of lemon	2	drachms.
" bergamot	8	"

Mix and filter.

New Mown Hay.

Extract of tonquin bean	32	ounces.
" geranium	16	"
" orange flowers	16	"
" rose flowers	16	"
" rose, triple	16	"
" jasmine	16	"

Mix and filter.

Royal Hunt Bouquet.

Esprit de rose, triple . .	16 ounces.
" neroli . . .	4 "
" acacia . . .	4 "
" fleur d'orange .	4 "
" musk . . .	4 "
" orris . . .	4 "
" tonquin . .	8 "
Oil of lemon zest . .	2 drachms.

Mix and filter.

Bouquet de Flore.

Esprit de rose " tubereuse " violet	from pomade, of each 16 ounces.
Extract of benzoin . .	1½ ounce.
Oil of bergamot . . .	2 ounces.
" lemon zest . .	4 drachms.
" orange zest . .	4 "

Mix and filter.

Guard's Bouquet.

Esprit de rose . . .	2 pints.
" neroli . . .	8 ounces.
Extract of vanilla . .	8 "
" orris . .	8 "
" musk . .	4 "
Oil of cloves . . .	30 drops.

Mix and filter.

Jockey Club Bouquet (*English*).

Extract of orris root . .	2 pounds.
Esprit de rose, triple . .	1 pound.
" " de pommade	1 "
Extrait de cassie	from pomade, of each 8 ounces.
" tubereuse	
" ambergris . .	8 ounces.
Oil of bergamot . . .	4 drachms.

Mix and filter.

Jockey Club Bouquet (*French*).

Esprit de rose, de pommade	16 ounces.
" tubereuse . .	16 "
" cassie . . .	8 "
" jasmin . .	12 "
Extrait de civet . . .	3 "

Mix and filter.

Japanese Perfume.

Extract of rose, triple .	8 ounces.
" vitivert . .	8 "
" patchouly . .	8 "
" cedar . .	8 "
" sandal . .	8 "
" vervain . .	4 "

Mix and filter.

Kew Garden Nosegay.

Esprit de neroli . . .	16 ounces.
" cassie	from pomade, of each 8 ounces.
" tubereuse	
" jasmin	
" geranium . .	8 ounces.
" musk . . .	3 "
" ambergris . .	3 "

Mix and filter.

Stolen Kisses.

Extract of jonquil . .	1 quart.
" orris . . .	1 "
" tonquin . .	1 pint.
" rose, triple .	1 "
" acacia . .	1 "
" civet . . .	¼ "
" ambergris . .	¼ "
Oil of citronella . . .	1 drachm.
" verbena . . .	30 drops.

Mix and filter.

Caprice de la Mode.

Extrait de jasmin . .	8 ounces.
" tubereuse . .	8 "
" cassie . .	8 "
" fleur d'orange .	8 "
Otto of almonds . . .	10 drops.
" nutmegs . . .	10 "
Extract of civet . . .	4 ounces.

Mix and filter.

May Flowers.

Extract of rose . . .	8	ounces.
" jasmine . .	8	"
" fleur d'orange .	8	"
" cassia . .	8	"
" vanilla . .	16	"
Oil of almonds . . .	15	drops.

Mix and filter.

Leap Year Bouquet.

Extrait de tubereuse . .	16	ounces.
" jasmin . .	16	"
" rose, triple .	8	"
" sandal . .	8	"
" vitivert . .	8	"
" patchouly . .	8	"
" verbena . .	2	"

Mix and filter.

Bouquet du Roi.

Extract of jasmine (from pomade)	16	ounces.
" violet "	16	"
" rose "	16	"
" vanilla . .	4	"
" vitivert . .	4	"
" musk . .	1	ounce.
" ambergris . .	1	"
Oil of bergamot . .	1	drachm.
" cloves . . .	1	ounce.

Mix and filter.

Isle of Wight Bouquet.

Extract of orris . . .	8	ounces.
" vitivert . .	4	"
" sandal . .	16	"
" rose . . .	8	"

Mix and filter.

Bouquet de la Reine.

Esprit de rose (from pomade)	16	ounces.
Extrait de violette "	16	"
" tubereuse . .	8	"
" fleur d'orange .	4	"
Oil of bergamot . . .	2	drachms.

Mix and filter.

Bouquet of all Nations.

Countries in which the odors are produced.			
Turkey . . .	Esprit de rose, triple	8	ounces.
Africa . . .	Extract of jasmine .	8	"
England . .	" lavender	4	"
France . . .	" tuberose	8	"
South America	" vanilla .	4	"
North "	" magnolia	4	"
Timor . . .	" sandal .	4	"
Italy	" violet .	16	"
Hindoostan .	" patchouly	4	"
Ceylon . . .	Oil of citronella .	1	drachm.
Sardinia . .	" lemon . .	2	drachms.
Tonquin . .	Extract of musk .	4	ounces.

Mix and filter.

Essence of Rondeletia.

Spirit at 75° . . .	1 gallon.
Oil of lavender . . .	2 ounces.
" cloves . . .	1 ounce.
" roses . . .	3 drachms.
" bergamot . . .	1 ounce.
Extract of musk . .	4 ounces.
" vanilla . .	4 "
" ambergris . .	4 "

Mix and filter.

Tulip Nosegay.

Extract of tuberose (from pomade)	16 ounces.
" violet "	16 "
" jasmine "	16 "
" rose . . .	8 "
" orris . . .	3 "
Oil of almonds . . .	3 drops.

Mix and filter.

West End Bouquet.

Extract of cassia . .	16 ounces.
" violet . .	16 "
" tuberose . .	16 "
" jasmine . .	16 "
Esprit de rose, triple . .	48 "
Extract of musk . .	8 "
" ambergris . .	8 "
Oil of bergamot . .	1 ounce.

Mix and filter.

Rifle Volunteer's Garland.

Rectified alcohol	. .	16 ounces.
Oil of neroli	. . .	2 drachms.
" rose	. . . .	2 "
" lavender	. . .	2 "
" bergamot	. . .	2 "
" cloves	. . .	8 drops.
Extract of orris	. . .	16 ounces.
" jasmine	. .	4 "
" cassia	. .	4 "
" musk	. .	2½ "
" ambergris	. .	2½ "

Mix and filter.

Yacht Club Bouquet.

Extract of sandal	. .	16 ounces.
" neroli	. .	16 "
" jasmine	. .	8 "
" rose, triple	.	8 "
" vanilla	. .	4 "
Flowers of benzoin	. .	2 drachms.

Mix and filter.

Violette des Bois.

Extract of violet	. .	16 ounces.
" orris	. . .	3 "
" cassia	. .	3 "
" rose (from pomade)		3 "
Oil of almonds	. . .	3 drops.

Mix and filter.

CHAPTER XVII.

PERFUMES FOR PASTES AND POMADES.

Parfum Amer à la Rose.

Oil of bitter almonds	2 ounces.
" bergamot	8 "
" cloves	1 ounce.
" geranium	5 ounces.

Mix. It is very fine for soaps and pastes for the hands.

Parfum d'Oeillet.

Alcohol	1 quart.
Extract of violet	4 ounces.
Oil of cloves	2 drachms.
Tincture of benzoin	4 "
" ambergris	1 drachm.

Mix and add—

Rose water	2 ounces.
Orange flower water	2 "

Filter several times

Parfum de Violette.

Alcohol	1 quart.
Orris root	1 pound.
Extract of cassia	8 ounces.

Macerate forty days, filter, and add—

Extract of jasmine	2 ounces.

Parfum d' Orange.

Alcohol	1 quart.
Oil of Portugal . . .	4 drachms.
" bergamot . .	2 "
Tincture of ambergris .	1 drachm.
Extract of orange flower .	8 ounces.

Mix well.

Parfum à la Verveine.

Alcohol	8 ounces.
Oil of vervain . . .	4 drachms.
" bergamot . .	2 "
Spirit of citronella . .	4 "

Mix well.

Eau Styptique de Myrte.

Alcohol	1 pint.
Oil of myrtle . . .	2 drachms.
Tannin	4 "
Tincture of catechu . .	8 "
Lavender water	1 pint.

Mix well, let it settle a few hours, and filter.

Parfum de Plaisir.

Citronella,	Marjoram,	Origanum,
Sweet basil,	Melilot,	Rosemary,
Hyssop,	Melisse,	Thyme,
Orris,	Mint,	Rose leaves.
Lavender,		

Take two handfuls of each; introduce them into an alembic which is filled two-thirds with water. Distil at a gentle heat. The distillate is introduced into an earthen jar, and left till next day. Then separate the oil from the water, and dissolve it in two or three quarts of rectified alcohol. Introduce this alcoholate into the alembic, and distil anew over a water bath.

Eau de Luce.

Rectified oil of amber .	4 drachms.
Mecca balsam . . .	½ drachm.
White soap . . .	½ "
Alcohol at 90° . . .	10 ounces.
Oil of lavender . . .	15 drops.

Dissolve the balsam and oil in the alcohol, add the soap, let it stand ten days, filter, and to the filtrate add—

Aqua ammonia . . . 8 ounces.

Shake well, and keep in well-corked bottles.

Eau de Melisse des Carmes.

This water is prepared with three ounces of each of the following substances:—

1. Coarsely-powdered cinnamon.
   " " cloves.
   " " nutmegs.
   Anise seed.
   Coriander seed.
   Dry lemon peel.

Macerate each of these substances separately for three days in one quart of alcohol at 58°, and distil separately over a water bath. The distillation is continued until the liquid passes drop by drop.

Distil afterwards in the same manner and the same proportion, after a maceration of three or four days, three ounces of the following plants:—

2. With one quart of alcohol at 58°.

Angelica . . .	all the plant.
Rosemary, Marjoram, Hyssop, Thyme, Sage,	Leaves and flowers without the stems.

Take some fresh melisse recently collected, mix it in the proportion of three ounces for one quart of alcohol, and distil it in the same manner after maceration. When all these preliminary preparations have been made, and each substance is in a separate bottle, mix them in three jars in the following proportions:—

Jar No. 1.

Alcoholate of	cinnamon .	3	quarts.
"	cloves . .	3	"
"	nutmegs .	3	"
"	anise . .	2	"
"	coriander .	3	"
"	lemon . .	8	"

Mix and keep.

Jar No. 2.

Alcoholate of angelica	10	quarts.
" rosemary	6	"
" marjoram	7	"
" hyssop	8	"
" thyme	7	"
" sage	15	"

Mix.

Jar No. 3.

Contains only the alcoholate of melisse.

When the eau de melisse des carmes is to be made, make the following mixture:—

From jar No. 1	5	quarts.
" jar No. 2	5	"
" jar No. 3	5¼	"

Mix, add three pints of water and six ounces of sugar, and distil over a water bath.

Another.

Fresh melisse flowers	24	ounces.
Fresh lemon peel	4	"
Cinnamon	2	"
Cloves	2	"
Nutmegs	2	"
Coriander	2	"
Angelica root	1	ounce.
Mint water	1	"

Macerate five days in four quarts of alcohol.

Distil off the spirituous part.

Another.

Fresh flowers of melisse .	13 ounces.
Angelica	2 "
Hyssop	1½ ounce.
Marjoram	1½ "
Rosemary	1 "
Cinnamon	1 "
Thyme	1½ "
Coriander	1½ "
Cloves	1 "
Nutmegs	1 "
Anise	4 drachms.
Lemon peel	1 ounce.
Alcohol at 58°	9 pints.

Macerate a few days, and distil over a water bath.

SECTION IX.

VINEGARS.

VINEGAR is a product obtained by subjecting to acetic fermentation wine, beer, or other alcoholic liquors. The acidification takes place at the expense of the alcohol, which experiences a complete transformation. The ancients knew that the production of vinegar could not be effected without the introduction of the air and some foreign matters contained in the liquors. But it is only by the experiments of Davy and Dæbereiner that we know exactly the part the air plays in this phenomenon. Davy first observed that platina black in contact with alcohol, became incandescent, and at the same time acetic acid is formed. Upon this fact Dæbereiner founded a scientific theory of the transformation of alcohol into acetic acid. He demonstrated that this transformation was effected by the absorption of oxygen from the air.

Toilet vinegars are made by impregnating this liquid with various perfumes and aromatics, such as lemon, vanilla, &c.

CHAPTER XVIII.

TOILET VINEGARS.

Lavender Vinegar.

Fresh flowers of lavender .	2 pounds.
White vinegar . . .	6 quarts.

Macerate two weeks and distil.

To the distillate add—

Tincture of benzoin . .	1 pound.

Distil again.

Rose Vinegar.

Pale roses	4 pounds.
White vinegar . . .	4 quarts.
Rhodium wood . . .	8 ounces.
Tincture of benzoin . .	8 "

Macerate two weeks and distil.

Rosemary Vinegar.

Flowers of rosemary . .	2 pounds.
Vinegar	4 quarts.

Infuse three weeks and distil.

Detersive Vinegar.

Narcissus bulbs . . .	6
Powdered nettle seeds .	1 ounce
Vinegar	1 quart.

Macerate for three days, express and filter.

Antiseptic Vinegar (of the Four Thieves).

Dried top of wormwood	.	12½ drachms.
" rosemary	.	12½ "
" sage	. .	12½ "
" mint	. .	12½ "
" rue	. .	12½ "
Dried flowers of lavender	.	2 ounces.
Garlic	. . . .	2 drachms.
Calamus	. . . .	2 "
Cinnamon	. . . .	2 "
Cloves	. . . .	2 "
Nutmegs	. . . .	2 "
Red vinegar	. . .	8 pounds.
Spirits of camphor	. .	4 drachms.

All these substances are coarsely powdered, and macerated for two weeks in the vinegar. Pass through a cloth, express, and distil. Add the camphorated alcohol to the distillate, and keep in ground-stoppered bottles.

Aromatic Vinegar of the Regent.

Alcohol at 90°	. . .	2 pounds.
Melisse water	. . .	1 pound.
Cologne "	. . .	1 "
Tincture of balsam of Tolu		3½ ounces.
" benzoin	. .	2 "
" musked amber		4 drachms.
Oil of lavender	. . .	2 ounces.
" cloves	. . .	1¼ drachm.
" cinnamon	. . .	1¼ "

After dissolving the oils with the alcohol, let them stand a few hours, and add—

Acetic acid	. . .	3½ ounces.

Color with archil, and filter until the liquid is perfectly clear.

Bully's Vinegar.

Water	. . . .	7 quarts.
Alcohol	. . . .	3½ "
Oil of bergamot	. . .	1 ounce.
" lemon	. . .	1 "
" Portugal	. . .	3 drachms.
" rosemary	. . .	6 "
" lavender	. . .	1 drachm.
" neroli	. . .	1 "
Alcoholate of melisse	. .	1 pound.

Macerate twenty-four hours, and add—

Tincture of benzoin	. .	2 ounces.
" Tolu	. .	2 "
" storax	. .	2 "
" cloves	. .	2 "

Stir, and add—

Distilled vinegar	. .	2 quarts.
Acetic acid	. . .	3 ounces.

Filter.

Toilet Vinegar (Sinfar).

Alcohol at 90° . . .	8	quarts.
White vinegar . . .	2	"
Cologne water . . .	1	pint.
Extract of benzoin . .	60	quarts.
" storax . .	60	"
Pure vinegar . . .	125	"
Oil of lavender . . .	45	"
" cinnamon . . .	4	"
" cloves . . .	4	"
Ammonia	4	"

Macerate for eight days the alcohol, lavender, cinnamon, and cloves, then add the cologne water, the vinegar, extracts, and the alkali. Color with archil, and filter.

Cosmetic Vinegar of the Hygienic Society.

Alcohol at 90° . . .	100	quarts.
Spirit of melisse . . .	15	"
" lavender . .	10	"
" rosemary . .	10	"
Oil of bergamot . . .	2	pounds.
" bitter orange . .	20	ounces.
" lemon . . .	13	"
" orange . . .	12	"
" neroli . . .	7	"
" mint . . .	5	"
" thyme . . .	5	"
" cloves . . .	2	"
" cinnamon . . .	1	ounce.
" vervain . . .	5	ounces.

Macerate the whole, and distil 126 quarts. Macerate one month in 42 quarts of this distillate 30 pounds orris and 4 pounds balsam of Tolu. Filter. Mix with the balance of the distillate, add 15 quarts of acetic acid at 80°, and, after twenty-four hours, filter.

Aromatic Vinegar.

Concentrated acetic acid .	8 ounces.
Oil of lavender	2 drachms.
" rosemary . . .	1 drachm.
" cloves . . .	1 "
" camphor . . .	1 ounce.

Dissolve the camphor in the acetic acid, then add the perfumes. After remaining together for a few days, with occasional agitation, it is to be filtered and bottled for use or sale.

Hygienic or Preventive Vinegar.

Brandy	1 pint.
Oil of cloves . . .	1 drachm.
" lavender . . .	1 "
" marjoram . . .	½ "
Gum benzoin . . .	1 ounce.

Macerate a few hours, and add—

Brown vinegar . . .	1 quart.

Strain and filter, if necessary.

Toilet Vinegar (à la Violette).

Extract of cassia	8 ounces.
" orris	4 "
Esprit de rose, triple	4 "
White vinegar	1 quart.

Cosmetic Vinegar (Piesse and Lubin).

Spirit	1 quart.
Gum benzoin	3 ounces.
Concentrated aromatic vinegar	1 ounce.
Balsam Peru	1 "
Otto neroli	1 drachm.
" nutmeg	½ "

Inexhaustible Salts for Smelling-Bottles.

Liquid ammonia	1 pint.
Otto of rosemary	1 drachm.
" lavender	1 "
" bergamot	½ "
" cloves	½ "

Mix the whole together by agitation in a very strong, and well-stoppered bottle. Used to fill smelling-bottles.

SECTION X.

MILKS AND LOTIONS.

Names given to certain cosmetic preparations which have the appearance of milk.

All these compounds are more or less injurious to the health of the skin, on account of the salts of lead or resins which enter into their composition.

CHAPTER XIX.

MILKS.

Aromatic Virginal Milk.

Benzoin	8 ounces.
Storax	4 "
Cyperus	1 ounce.
Cinnamon	1 "
Nutmeg	5 drachms.
Ambrette	10 "
Tincture of musk	2 "

All these substances are coarsely powdered, and digested for three weeks in—

Alcohol at 93°	. . .	1 gallon.

Stir every day, and filter.

Four drops of this alcoholate, poured into a glass of water, renders the liquid mucky, because water will not dissolve the resins and essential oils, which are held in a state of suspension in the mixture.

Milk of Almonds.

Sweet almonds	. . .	1 pound.
Bitter "	. . .	2 ounces.

Grind in a marble mortar until the whole is reduced to a homogeneous mass. In a porcelain dish and over a water bath melt—

Spermaceti	. . .	1 ounce.
White wax	. . .	½ "
Almond oil	. . .	1 "
White soap	. . .	1 "

When melted, take from the mortar three-quarters of the almonds and pour on the melted grease; stir quickly. Then add little by little the almonds, triturating all the time. When the mass forms a homogeneous paste, pour on it, little by little, stirring all the time—

Rose water	. . .	4 pints.
Spirit of roses	. . .	10 ounces.

A milky emulsion is obtained, which is passed through a cotton cloth under pressure, and is then poured into vials. More perfume may be given by adding a little oil of roses.

Cucumber Milk.

Operate as above, but instead of rose water, pour into the mortar two quarts of juice of cucumbers, and ten ounces of rectified alcohol.

Milk of Roses.

Almonds (blanched) . .	8 ounces.
Rose water . . .	1 quart.
Alcohol at 75° . . .	4 ounces.
Oil of rose	1 drachm.
White wax, spermaceti, oil-soap, each . . .	½ ounce.

Cut the soap into shavings; heat it in a vessel over a water bath; add to it two or three ounces of rose water. When melted add the wax and spermaceti, and melt slowly. Beat the almonds well in a mortar, allowing the rose water to trickle into the mass by degrees. When the emulsion of almonds is finished strain it through bleached muslin.

The saponaceous mixture is then poured into the mortar, and is carefully blended with the emulsion. As the last of the soap mixture is added, the spirit in which the otto of roses has been previously dissolved is gradually poured in. When the whole is well mixed it is strained.

Lait du Japon.

Oil of sweet almonds	. .	4 ounces.
" tartar	. . .	2 "
" rhodium	. . .	2 drachms.
" jonquil	. . .	1 drachm.

Mix and filter.

CHAPTER XX.

LOTIONS.

Cosmetic Lotion of Alibert.

Rose water	. . .	1 quart.
Amygdaline soap	. .	3 drachms.
Cucumber pomade	. .	3 ounces.

The soap is ground with the pomade, and the water is added little by little. Rose water may be substituted by any other perfume.

Excellent for the skin.

Cosmetic Water.

Bitter almonds	. . .	10 ounces.
Water	. . . .	5 pints.

Distil so as to obtain three pints of liquid, and add—

Spirituous water of roses	.	2 pounds.
Odoriferous honey water	.	4 "

For use dissolve two spoonfuls in a tumbler of water. Very good for the skin.

Lotion of Gowland.

Bitter almonds . . .	3 ounces.
Distilled water . . .	16 "
Corrosive sublimate . .	1½ grain.
Sal ammoniac . . .	2 drachms.
Alcohol	4 "
Cherry-laurel water . .	4 "

Grind the almonds with the water, and pass through a cloth. Dissolve the salts in the cherry-laurel water and the alcohol. Mix the two solutions. The lotion is very much used in England as a cosmetic; it is principally employed as a remedy for eczema.[1]

Lotion for Freckles.

Borax	3 grains.
Rose water	5 drachms.
Orange flower water . .	5 "

Wash the skin with the solution once or twice a day.

Sulphuretted Ammoniacal Lotion.

Concentrated solution of sulphide of potassium . .	1 ounce.
Sulphydrate of ammonia .	½ drachm.

Mix the two. Wash the affected parts with the preparation.

[1] On account of the mercury it contains, it is a very unsafe article for general use.

Astringent Lotion.

Plantain water . . .	5 ounces.
Tannin	1¼ drachm.
Aromatic tincture . .	6 drachms.

Rub the tannin, moistening it by degrees with the tincture, then pour in the water, and when the whole is dissolved pass through a cloth.

Another.

Sulphate of zinc . .	1 drachm.
" alumina . .	1 "
Plantain water . . .	1 pint.

Proceed as above.

Cosmetic Lotion.

Bitter almonds . . .	10 ounces.
Water	2 quarts.

Distil over a water-bath so as to obtain one quart; then add:—

Odoriferous honey-water .	8 ounces.
Rosat vinegar . . .	16 "

Aromatize with

Oil of bergamot . . .	4 drachms.
Tincture of Tolu . .	2½ "

Use, diluting a teaspoonful with a tumbler of water, as a wash for the skin.

Another.

Animal soap . . .	½ ounce.
Cucumber pomade . .	3½ ounces.
Cherry-laurel water . .	1 quart.

Triturate the soap with the pomade, add the water by degrees, and rub until a homogeneous liquid is obtained.

This cosmetic renders the skin very bright and soft.

Glycerine Lotion.

Orange-flower water . .	1 gallon.
Glycerine	8 ounces.
Borax	1 ounce.

Dissolve. Filter.

An excellent cosmetic.

SECTION XI.

DENTIFRICES.

PREPARATIONS used not only to cleanse the teeth, but also to strengthen the gums. Great care must be taken in the selection of the materials used, so as to avoid the destruction of the enamel of the teeth. These preparations are sold in three different forms: 1. Washes or fluids; 2. Pastes; 3. Powders.

CHAPTER XXI.

WATERS.

Botot's Dental Fluid.

Cloves . . . . 2 drachms.
Cinnamon . . . . 2 "
Aniseed . . . . 1 ounce.
Cochineal . . . . 2½ drachms.
Brandy . . . . 29 ounces.

Macerate two weeks in the brandy, filter, and add

Oil of mint . . . 1¼ drachm.

O'Meara's Dental Fluid.

Vetiver	1 drachm.
Pyrethrum	4 drachms.
Cloves	4½ grains.
Orris	1½ drachm.
Coriander	1½ "
Alkanet	1½ "
Oil of mint	12 drops.
" bergamot	6 "
Alcohol at 90°	2 ounces.

Macerate for one week and filter.

Delabarre's Dental Fluid.

Alcohol	4 ounces.
Oil of mint	20 drops.
" rose	8 "
Cochineal	8 grains.
Cream tartar	9½ "

Macerate for three days and filter.

Greenough's Dentifrice Tincture.

Bitter almonds	2 ounces.
Brazil wood	½ ounce.
Fir-tree buds	½ "
Orris root	2 drachms.
Cochineal	1 drachm.
Binoxalate of potash	1 "
Alcohol	1 quart.

Macerate three weeks in the alcohol, filter, and add—

Spirit of cochlearia . .	2 ounces.
Oil of peppermint . .	½ ounce.

Jackson's Balsamic Dental Fluid.

Orange zest . . .	2 ounces.
Lemon zest . . .	2 "
Pomegranate bark . .	2 "
Angelica root . . .	2 "
Guaiacum	5 "
Pyrethrum	6 "
Benzoin	2 "
Tolu	2 "
Clove	2 "
Cinnamon	½ ounce.
Vanilla	½ "
Myrrh	½ "
Alcohol	2 quarts.

Macerate one week and filter, and add to the filtrate—

Tincture of cochlearia .	1 pint.
Oil of peppermint . .	6 drachms.

Dental Elixir (Desirabode).

Guaiacum brandy . .	6 ounces.
Spirituous vulnerary water.	6 "
An essential oil . . .	4 drops.

Two or three drops are sufficient to aromatize a glass of water.

Aromatic Elixir (*Lefoulon*).

Tincture of vanilla	. .	½ ounce.
" pyrethrum	. .	4 ounces.
Alcoholate of mint	. .	1 ounce.
" rosemary	.	1 "
" roses	. .	2 ounces.

Mix. A few drops in a glass of water to rinse the mouth.

Dental Tincture of Pyrethrum.

Cinnamon	. . . . .	2½ drachms.
Coriander	. . . . .	2½ "
Cochineal	. . . . .	½ drachm.
Cloves	. . . .	1¼ "
Mace	. . . . . .	1¼ "
Sal ammoniac	. . .	¼ "
Alcoholate of pyrethrum	.	3 pints.

Macerate two weeks and filter; add to the filtrate—

Oil of peppermint	. .	1½ drachm.
" lemon	. . .	¾ "
" thyme	. . .	½ "
" anise	. . .	1 "
" lavender	. . .	½ "
Tincture of ambergris	.	½ "

Stir well, let it stand a few hours, and filter.

Treasure of the Mouth.

Alcoholate of cochlearia	.	7 ounces.
" lavender	.	3½ "
" peppermint	.	3½ "
" lemon .	.	3½ "

Mix. A teaspoonful in a glass of water to rinse the mouth.

Vinegar of Lavender.

Strong vinegar . .	.	4 ounces.
Alcoholate of lavender	.	4 "

Mix. A teaspoonful in a glass of water. Used as an odontalgic.

Odontalgic Elixir (Ancelot).

Alcoholate of rosemary	.	3 ounces.
Pyrethrum (root) .	.	3 drachms.

Macerate three days, filter. Mix with four times its weight of water to rinse the mouth.

Odontalgic Elixir (Leroy).

Guaiacum . . .	.	4 drachms.
Pyrethrum . . .	.	1 drachm.
Nutmegs . . .	.	1 "
Cloves . . .	.	½ "
Oil of rosemary . .	.	10 drops.
" bergamot . .	.	4 "
Alcohol at 70° . .	.	3½ ounces.

Macerate eight days; filter. A teaspoonful in a glass of water to rinse the mouth.

Odontalgic Elixir (*Desforges*).

Coarsely-ground cinchona bark	4 ounces.
" " guaiacum .	5 "
Pyrethrum	4 "
Cloves	5 drachms.
Orange peel	2 "
Saffron	½ drachm.
Benzoin	2 drachms.

Macerate for five or six days in—

Alcohol at 80°	4 pints.

Filter and bottle for use. One or two teaspoonfuls in a glass of water to rinse the mouth.

Odontalgic Gargle (*Plenck*).

Distilled lavender water .	2 ounces.
" vinegar	2 "
Pyrethrum (root) . . .	2 drachms.
Hydrochlorate of ammonia	¼ drachm.
Extract of opium . . .	1½ grain.

Digest a few days and filter. Use in nervous and rheumatic toothache.

Odontalgic Elixir (*Bories*).

Pyrethrum	1 ounce.
Spirit of lavender . . .	16 ounces.
Sal ammoniac	½ drachm.

Macerate twenty-four hours, and filter.

Odontalgic Spirit (Boerhaave).

Alcohol	2 drachms.
Camphor	1 drachm.
Opium	3¾ grains.
Oil of cloves . . .	20 drops.

Mix. To be introduced into the cavity of the tooth on a pledget of raw cotton.

Odontalgic Mixture (Cadet).

Ether	1¼ drachm.
Laudanum	1¼ "
Balsam of the commandeur	1¼ "
Oil of cloves . . .	1¼ "

Apply to the tooth on a little cotton-wool.

Odontalgic Mixture (Oudet).

Acetic ether . . .	2½ drachms.
Laudanum	2½ "
Oil of cloves . . .	2½ "

Apply to the tooth by means of a little cotton.

Odontalgic Collyrium (Oudet).

Tincture of Para cress* .	2 ounces.
Alcoholate of peppermint .	2 "
Alcohol at 56° . . .	3½ "
Creasote	½ drachm.

Moisten a little cotton with it, and apply to the tooth.

* Tropæolus magus ; Indian cress.

Odontalgic Essence (*Meyer*).

Camphor	$6\frac{1}{4}$ grains.
Oil of cloves . . .	20 drops.
" turpentine . .	20 "
" cajeput . . .	20 "

Dissolvè. One or two drops in the tooth, on cotton-wool.

Odontalgic Liniment (*Chapman*).

Camphor	1 drachm.
Spirit of turpentine . .	4 drachms.

Dissolve. A few drops on the tooth, or rubbed on the face over the tooth.

Anti-Odontalgic Mixture (*Toirac*).

Acetate of lead . . .	$\frac{1}{4}$ drachm.
Sulphate of zinc . . .	$\frac{1}{4}$ "
Tincture of opium . .	$\frac{1}{2}$ "

One drop in the tooth.

Anti-Odontalgic Topic (*Handel*).

Extract of hyoscyamus .	1 drachm.
Opium	$\frac{1}{2}$ "
Extract of belladonna . .	$\frac{1}{2}$ "
Camphor	$4\frac{3}{4}$ grains.
Tincture of Spanish flies .	3 drops.
Oil of cajeput . . .	8 "

To be introduced into the cavity of the tooth.

Acetic Alum Paste.

Powdered alum	. . .	2½ drachms.
Gum Arabic	. . .	2½ "
Acetic ether	. . .	½ drachm.

Make a paste with a sufficient quantity of mucilage, and introduce a small pellet into the cavity of the tooth.

CHAPTER XXII.

DENTIFRICE POWDERS.

Delestre's Powder.

Calcined magnesia . .	3 drachms.
Calisaya bark . . .	3 "
Powdered rhatany . .	½ drachm.
" tobacco . .	½ "
" pyrethrum . .	10 grains.
" calcined alum .	10 "
Soot	4 "

Mix, pass through a fine sieve, and aromatize with oil of mint.

Mialhe's Powder.

Powdered sugar of milk .	14 ounces.
Pure tannin . . .	1½ drachm.
Carminated lake . .	1 "
Oil of mint . . .	2 drachms.
" anise . . .	2 "
" orange flower . .	1 drachm.

Mix.

Charcoal Tooth-Powder.

Powdered vegetable charcoal	2 ounces.
" calisaya bark .	1 ounce.
Carbonate of magnesia .	2 drachms.

Mix. Aromatize with a few drops of any essential oil.

Another.

Calcined magnesia . .	4 drachms.
Sulphate of quinia . .	8 grains.
Liquid carmine . . .	8 "
Oil of mint . . .	4 drops.

Toirac's Powder.

Precipitated chalk . .	1 drachm.
Magnesia	2 drachms.
Powdered sugar . . .	1 drachm.
Bitartrate of potash . .	¼ "
Oil of mint . . .	¼ "

French Codex Powder.

Armenian bole . . .	3 ounces.
Coral	3 "
Bones	3 "
Resin of dragon's blood .	1½ ounce.
Cochineal	3 drachms.
Cream of tartar . . .	5 ounces.
Powdered cinnamon . .	1 ounce.
" cloves . .	1 drachm.

Mix well in a mortar, and pass through a hair sieve.

Another.

Powdered bones . . .	2¾ ounces.
" orris root . .	2¾ "
" cream of tartar .	2 "
" cloves . .	5 drachms.
Carminated lake . .	2¾ ounces.

Mix well, and pass through a fine sieve.

Charlat's Powder.

Cream of tartar . . .	5 ounces.
Calcined alum . . .	2½ drachms.
Cochineal	2 "

Reduce to a fine powder, and aromatize with

Oil of roses . . .	5 drops.

Charcoal and Magnesia Powder.

Charcoal	7 ounces
Magnesia	2½ drachms.

Powder carefully, and aromatize with

Oil of mint . . .	15 drops.

Deschamp's Powder.

Powdered talc . . .	4 ounces.
Bicarbonate of soda . .	1 ounce.
Carmine	4½ grains.
Oil of mint . . .	15 drops.

Mix.

Maury's Powder.

Charcoal	8 ounces.
Cinchona bark . . .	4 "
Sugar	8 "
Oil of mint	4 drachms.
" cinnamon . . .	2 "
Tincture of ambergris .	½ drachm.

Reduce to a fine powder.

English Powder.

Precipitated chalk . . .	$\frac{3}{4}$ drachm.
Camphor	$\frac{1}{4}$ "

Mix.

Jamet's Powder.

Orris root	16 ounces.
Magnesia	4 "
Pumice stone	8 "
Bones	8 "
Sulphate of quinia . . .	4 "
Cascarilla	1 ounce.
Sugar of milk	16 ounces.
Oil of mint	1 ounce.
" cinnamon	2 drachms.
" neroli	1 drachm.
Tincture of ambergris . . .	1 "

Reduce to a very fine powder, and pass through a hair sieve.

Piesse's Farina Powder.

Burnt horn	2 pounds.
Orris root	2 "
Carmine	1 drachm.
Powdered sugar	8 ounces.
Oil of neroli	$\frac{1}{2}$ drachm.
" lemon	2 drachms.
" bergamot	2 "
" orange peel . . .	2 "
" rosemary	1 drachm.

CHAPTER XXIII.

OPIATES.

THE uses of opiates are the same as powders; they differ from the latter only by the addition of honey or syrup. To prepare them, melt one pound of good honey; skim it carefully; add seven ounces of syrup of sugar; stir the mixture, and pour into a marble mortar, into which throw the prepared powder a little at a time, rubbing until completely incorporated and perfectly homogeneous. Aromatize with essences of cinnamon, cloves, mint, etc. When a half-liquid opiate is obtained pour into jars.

Red Tooth Opiate.

Powdered coral . . .	4 ounces.
Bones	1 ounce.
Cream of tartar . . .	2 ounces.
Cochineal	1 ounce.
Alum	½ drachm.
White honey . . .	10 ounces.

Grind the cochineal with the alum and a little water; add the honey—then the other ingredients; lastly, aromatize with oil of mint.

Pelletier's Odontine.

Butter of coco Carbonate of magnesia Clay	undetermined proportions.

Aromatize with oil of mint.

White Tooth Opiate.

White honey . . .	8 ounces.
Powdered orris . . .	5 "
Sal ammoniac . . .	1 ounce.
Cream of tartar . . .	1 "
Syrup of peppermint . .	1 "

Triturate in a marble mortar, and add—

Tincture of cinnamon .	2 drachms.
" cloves . .	2 "
" vanilla . .	2 "
Oil of cloves . . .	½ drachm.

Desforge's Tooth Opiate.

Powdered coral . . .	5 ounces.
" cream tartar .	1 ounce.
" bones . . .	5 drachms.
" cochineal . .	¾ drachm.
White honey . .	6 ounces.

Opiate Tooth Paste.

Honey	8 ounces.
Chalk	8 "
Orris	8 "
Carmine	2 drachms.
Oil of cloves . . .	½ drachm.
" nutmeg . . .	½ "
" rose	½ "

Syrup enough to form a paste.

SECTION XII.

COSMETIC PASTES—POWDERS—TROCHES—SACHETS.

CHAPTER XXIV.

PASTES.

Almond Paste.

Bitter almonds blanched and ground	1½ pound.
Rose water	1½ pint.
Alcohol at 60° above proof	1 pound.
Oil of bergamot . . .	3 ounces.

Place the ground almonds and one pint of the rose water in a stewpan. With a slow and steady heat cook the almonds until they become pasty, constantly stirring the mixture, otherwise the almonds will be burnt to the bottom of the pan and impart to the whole an empyreumatic odor. When the almonds are nearly cooked, the remaining rose water is added; finally the paste is put into a mortar and well rubbed; the perfume and spirit are then added. Before potting this paste it should be passed through a sieve.

Other pastes, such as the *pate de pistache*, *pate*

de cocos, *pate de guimauve*, etc., are prepared in the same manner.

Almond Meal.

Ground almonds	. .	1 pound.
Wheat flour	. . .	1 "
Orris-root powder	. .	4 ounces.
Oil of lemon	. . .	½ ounce.
" almonds	. . .	¼ drachm.

Pistachio Nut Meal.

Pistachio nuts	. . .	1 pound.
Orris powder	. . .	1 "
Oil of neroli	. . .	1 drachm.
" lemons	. . .	4 drachms.

Pound well together and pass through a fine sieve.

Other meals can be prepared in the same manner.

Almond Paste for the Hands.

Almond meal	. . .	12 ounces.
Rice flour	. . . .	4 "
Orris powder	. . .	4 "
Weak solution of soda	.	3½ "
Spermaceti	. . .	1 ounce.
Oil of bitter almonds	. .	5 ounces.
Rose water	. . . .	5 "

Melt the spermaceti in the oil of almonds; heat so as to bring the mixture to the consistency of cold cream, adding as much rose water as it will absorb. Pour into a marble mortar and add the orris powder and the flower of almonds or rice previously mixed; triturate well, moistening them from time to time with rose water and the solution of soda. When well mixed add—

Oil of lavender . . .	½ drachm.
" cloves . . .	½ "
" rhodium . . .	1 "

Beat until a very homogeneous paste is obtained.

Paté called Amandine Faquer.

Honey	6 ounces.
White potash soap . .	3 "
Almond oil . . .	2 pounds.
Pistachio milk . . .	4 ounces.
Five yelks of eggs.	

Melt the soap in the oil, stirring all the time; run into a mortar and beat, pouring in the milk of pistachio by degrees. When the mass is reduced to a homogeneous half fluid paste, add—

Oil of bitter almonds . .	½ drachm.

Then beat until well incorporated.

Paté à la Vanille.

Almond meal . . .	1 pound.
Tincture of vanilla . .	$1\frac{1}{4}$ drachm.
" Peru . .	$\frac{1}{2}$ " .
" Tolu . .	$\frac{1}{2}$ "
Six yelks of eggs beaten in rose water . . .	8 ounces.

Mix the almond meal with the rose water, and the yelks of eggs; incorporate the tinctures, triturating all the time. Add a little rose water if the paste is too thick, and lastly pour in one ounce of tincture of vanilla amber; heat until a homogeneous paste is obtained.

Paté d'Amande with Honey.

Bitter almond meal . .	6 ounces.
" " oil . .	$3\frac{1}{2}$ "
Honey	12 "
Eight yelks of eggs	
Subcarbonate of soda dissolved in rose water .	1 ounce.

Triturate in a mortar the meal, oil, and honey. Before adding the yelks, beat with them a little oil of bitter almonds; incorporate and beat well; add by small portions two ounces oil of bitter almonds; triturate for half an hour, until the paste does not attach itself to the mortar.

Paste of Horsechestnuts.

Horsechestnut meal . .	1 pound.
Oil of bitter almonds .	1 "
Miel rosat (honey of roses) .	13½ ounces.
White soap . . .	4 "
Twelve yelks of eggs	

Dissolve the soap in a sufficient quantity of rose water; add the honey and the oil; when the whole is dissolved, pour into a mortar, then throw the meal into it by small portions; when the paste is well beaten and homogeneous, perfume according to taste.

Transparent Paste.

Starch	5 ounces.
Castor oil	7 "
Potash soap . . .	7 "
Alcohol	14 "

Paté de Fraises for the Skin.

Fresh strawberries . .	4 ounces.
Gum tragacanth . .	¾ drachm.
Violet powder . . .	1 ounce.

Make a mucilage with distilled water and the gum.

Grind the strawberries in a mortar, throw in the violet powder and beat well to mix, pour in the mucilage little by little, and triturate until a half liquid homogeneous paste is obtained.

This preparation is to be prepared extemporaneously. It will not keep.

Olivine.

Powdered gum acacia . .	2 ounces.
Honey	6 "
Yelks of eggs	5
White soft soap . . .	3 ounces.
Olive oil	2 pounds.
Oil of bergamot . .	1 ounce.
" lemon	1 "
" clove	4 drachms.
" thyme and cassia, each	½ drachm.

Rub the gum and honey together until incorporated, then add the soap and eggs. Having mixed the perfumes with the olive oil, beat well.

CHAPTER XXV.

POWDERS.

THE powder used in perfumery is nothing but starch pulverized and passed through a fine sieve. When it has been moistened with alcohol, before powdering, it forms a lighter product called *purified powder with alcohol.*

Colored powders are prepared by different processes, sometimes burning the ordinary powder which then assumes a color more or less dark, sometimes by mixing it with powdered roots of odoriferous plants.

Absorbing Powder for Sweating of the Head.

Horsebean meal	. .	8 ounces.
White bean "	. .	8 "
Powder of staphisagria	.	3½ "

Mix.

Powder for Sweating of the Feet.

Carbonate of magnesia	.	3½ ounces.
Powdered calcined alum	.	1 ounce.
Orris root .	. . . .	3½ ounces.
Powdered cloves	. .	¼ drachm.

Mix.

Powder for the Skin.

Rye flour	8 ounces.
Melilot powder . . .	8 "
Violet " . . .	$2\frac{1}{2}$ "

With distilled water forms a paste which is applied at night to the face.

Cosmetic Powder for the Hands.

Bitter almond meal . .	1 pound.
Rice flour	8 ounces.
Sal soda in powder . .	1 ounce.
Oil of lavender . . .	2 drachms.

Mix.

Another.

Sweet almonds . . .	12 ounces.
Bitter " . . .	8 "
Rye flour	8 "
Bean "	16 "
Soap	19 "
Oil of Portugal . . .	2 drachms.

Mix.

Another.

Horsechestnut meal . .	16 ounces.
Bitter almond " . .	12 "
Orris root	1 ounce.
Carbonate of potash . .	$1\frac{3}{4}$ drachm.
Oil of bergamot . . .	1 "

Another.

Powdered soap . . .	12 ounces.
Carbonate of potash . .	2 "
Horse-chestnut meal . .	24 "
Bitter almond " . .	8 "
Oil of lemon . . .	½ drachm.
" cloves . . .	¼ "
" bergamot . .	¾ "
Powdered sugar . .	5 drachms.

Poudre d'Ambre Composée.

Cinnamon	½ drachm.
Cloves	¾ "
Mace	¾ "
Nutmegs	½ "
Galanga	½ "
Sassafras	½ "
Aloes	¾ "
Sandal	¾ "
Cardamom seed . . .	½ "
Zedoary	½ "
Lemon peel . . .	½ "
Amber	¼ "

Reduce to powder and pass through a fine sieve.

Fumigating Powder.

Incense	1 drachm.
Mastic	1 "
Powdered lavender . .	1 "
Cascarilla	½ "
Cloves	½ "
Cinnamon	¼ "
Benzoin	1¼ "
Myrrh	1 "

Powder together and pass through a sieve. Throw a little on a hot shovel to perfume an apartment.

Another, called Perfume of the Prince Kouratken.

Musk	1½ grain.
Benzoin	1 drachm.
Cascarilla	1 "
Storax	4 drachms.
Orris	4 "
Cloves	3 "
Cinnamon	3 "
Red roses	3 "
Flowers of lavender . .	6 "
" pomegranate .	6 "
Myrrh	1 drachm.
Mace	1 "
Oil of bergamot . . .	2½ drachms.
" clove	2½ "
" cinnamon . . .	2½ "
" geranium . . .	2½ "

Mix the whole in a fine powder. It is used as the last, and also for filling sachets.

Powder for Sachets.

Red roses	1 ounce.
Sandal	1 "
Cardamom	1 "
Cinnamon	½ "
Cloves	½ "
Saffron	2 drachms.
Anise	1 ounce.
Fennel	1 "
Orris	1 "

Rub together in a mortar, and pass through a sieve.

Poudre Fumigatoire (English).

Galbanum	1 ounce.
Benzoin	1 "
Myrrh	1 "
Cascarilla	½ "
Storax	2½ drachms.
Juniper	4 "

Make a powder which is thrown on lighted coals to perfume apartments.

Poudre à la Rose for Sachets.

Red roses	8 ounces.
Pale roses	8 "
Rhodium wood . . .	4 "
Ambrette	½ ounce.

Make a powder which is perfumed with

Oil of rose	6 drops.
" rhodium . . .	6 "
" geranium . . .	10 "

Pass through a sieve to fill sachets.

Poudre à la Vanille.

Vanilla, cut very fine . .	4 ounces.
Storax	4 "
Cloves	½ ounce.
Benzoin	4 ounces.
Rhodium wood . . .	4 "

Powder in a mortar and perfume with

Tincture of vanilla . .	½ drachm.
" musk . .	¼ "

Pass through a sieve to fill sachets.

Poudre au Portugal.

Dry orange peel . . .	14 ounces.
Cloves	½ drachm.
Storax	2 ounces.
Benzoin	2 "
Ambrette	1 ounce.
Ambergris . . .	¼ "

Powder, pass through a sieve to fill sachets.

Sachets of Eastern Women.

Orris	. . . . .	4 ounces.
Calamus aromaticus	. .	4 "
Sandal	. . . . .	$1\frac{1}{2}$ ounce.
Rhodium wood	. . .	$1\frac{1}{2}$ "
Cloves	. . . . .	1 "
Cinnamon	. . . .	1 "
Benzoin	. . . . .	6 drachms.
Myrrh	. . . . .	6 "
Green bergamots dried	.	4 ounces.
Powdered musk rose.	.	4 "
Ambergris	. . .	2 drachms.

Powder and pass through a sieve.

Another.

Powdered red and pale roses		8 ounces.
" cloves	. .	4 "
" nutmegs	. .	4 "
Orris and sandal	. .	8 "

Sachet au Chypre.

Ground rose-wood	. .	1 pound.
" cedar	. . .	1 "
" sandal	. . .	1 "
Oil of rose-wood	. .	3 drachms.

Mix and sift.

Frangipanni Sachet.

Powdered orris root . .	3 pounds.
" vitivert . .	4 ounces.
" sandal wood .	4 "
Oil of neroli . . .	1 drachm.
" rose	1 "
" sandal . . .	1 "
Ground musk . . .	1 ounce.
" civet . . .	2 drachms.

Marechale Sachet.

Powdered santal wood .	8 ounces.
" orris root . .	8 "
" rose leaves . .	4 "
" cloves . .	4 "
" cinnamon bark .	4 "
" musk . . .	½ drachm.

Millefleur Sachet.

Powdered lavender flowers	1 pound.
" orris . . .	1 "
" rose leaves .	1 "
Benzoin	1 "
Tonquin	4 ounces.
Vanilla	4 "
Sandal	4 "
Musk and civet, each . .	2 drachms.
Powdered cloves . . .	4 ounces.
Cinnamon	2 "
Allspice	2 "

Patchouly Sachet.

Powdered patchouly . .	1 pound.
Oil of patchouly . . .	¼ drachm.

Vervain Sachet.

Dry powdered lemon peel .	1 pound.
Lemon thyme . . .	4 ounces.
Oil of lemon grass . .	1 drachm.
" lemon peel . .	4 drachms.
" bergamot . . .	1 ounce.

CHAPTER XXVI.

CASSOLETTES.—POT POURRI.—TROCHISTS PASTILS.

Cassolettes are vessels made of fine clay, porcelain, or metal provided with a lid pierced with small holes. Cassolettes are filled with different perfumes, and when heated, the odor escapes through the holes and perfumes the apartment.

Cassolette du Serail.

Storax	4 drachms.
Benzoin	2 "
Mecca balsam	2 "
Cloves	¾ drachm.
Sandal	1 "
Amber	¼ "

Powder.

Cassolette à l'Ambre.

Black amber	4 pounds.
Rose powder	2 "
Benzoin	1 ounce.
Oil of rose	½ "
Gum tragacanth	½ "
Oil of sandal	few drops.

Powder.

POT POURRI is composed of a number of flowers, roots, aromatics, and other odoriferous substances, which are mixed in a large earthen jar and moistened with salt water.

The following is said to have been invented by Criton the Athenian, and was used in the lustral water in the temples of Aphrodite at Corinth:—

Orange flowers	1 pound.
Musk roses	1 "
Red pinks	7 ounces.
Marjoram	3½ "
Thyme	1 ounce.
Lavender	1 "
Rosemary	1 "
Melilot	1 "
Hyssop	1 "
Mint	1 "
Camomile	1 "
Laurel	10 leaves.
Jasmine flowers . . .	4 ounces.
Lemon peel . . .	4 "
Small green oranges . .	4 "
Kitchen salt	16 "

Introduce the whole into the jar, allowing it one month to macerate, stirring twice a day. After this time add—

Powdered orris . . .	10 ounces.
Benzoin	2 "
Cloves	2 "
Coriander	2 "
Storax	1 ounce.
Calamus aromaticus . .	1 "
Ambergris	1 "

Stir well.

Another.

Orange flower . . .	1 pound.
Red roses	8 ounces.
Lavender	8 "
Marjoram	4 "
Myrtle	2½ "
Red pinks	2 "
Cloves	2 drachms.
Nutmegs	2 "
Laurel	10 leaves.
Salt water	1 quart.

Macerate twenty days, stirring twice every day, then add—

Powder of chypre . .	1 ounce.
" orris . . .	1 "

PASTILLES.

Trochistes Odorants du Serail.

Benzoin	2 drachms.
Storax	1 drachm.
Labdanum	1 "

Orris	1 drachm.
Nutmegs	1 "
Rosemary	1 "
Sandal	1 "
Calamus aromaticus . .	1 "
Cloves	½ "
Cubebs	½ "

Grind these substances together in a mortar, adding gum tragacanth dissolved in a sufficient quantity of rose water, then add—

Civet	12½ grains.
Amber	4 drachms.
Musk	12½ grains.

Reduce the whole to a homogeneous paste, then add 20 drops of oil of cinnamon, stir and make in troches.

They are used in sachets, furnitures, cloth, pockets, etc.; they impart to them a very agreeable perfume.

Aromatic Trochists in Stick.

Cinnamon	1 drachm.
Cascarilla	1 "
Cloves	1 "
Succinum	2 drachms.
Vanilla	½ drachm.
Storax	1 "
Benzoin	1 "
Musk	1 grain.
Ambergris	1 "

Reduce to powder and add—

Balsam of Peru . . .	¼ drachm.
" Tolu . . .	½ "
" Mecca . .	¾ "

Moisten with a little rose water, so as to make a paste, which is rolled in sticks from four to five inches in length. Then they are dried in a slow oven or in the sun. Used to perfume apartments.

Cloux Fumants.

Gum benzoin	4 drachms.
Storax	1 drachm.
Balsam Peru . . .	2 drachms.
Cascarilla	1 drachm.
Cloves	½ "
Powdered charcoal . .	10 drachms.
Nitrate of potash . .	1 drachm.

Reduce to powder, and add—

Tincture of ambergris .	½ drachm.

Dissolve the nitrate of potash in a little warm gum-water and pour in the powder, which is well stirred, so as to make a paste. With this paste make cloues, pastilles, cardles, etc., which are dried in the oven.

Cloux Fumants du Serail.

Benzoin	2 ounces.
Balsam Tolu . . .	4 drachms.
Labdanum	1 drachm.
Sandal	4 drachms.

Light charcoal . . .	6 ounces.
Nitrate of potash . .	2 "
Mucilage of gum tragacanth	2 "

Proceed as in the above.

Pastils are little lozenges of different shapes and composed of sufficient substances which are used to perfume the air of a room by burning. They are prepared either by making a soft paste with sugar and mucilage, then adding the aromatics, etc.; the paste is then moulded into the shapes required.

Pastilles à la Rose.

Pale roses	4 ounces.
Rhodium wood . . .	8 "
Oil of roses . . .	½ drachm.
Powdered charcoal . .	4 ounces.
Nitrate of potash . .	1 drachm.

Pastilles des Indes.

Sandal	4 ounces.
Aloes wood . . .	4 "
Cinnamon	4 "
Rhodium wood . . .	2 "
Cedar wood . . .	2 "
Cloves	1 ounce.
Myrrh	2 ounces.
Vanilla	1 ounce.
Amber	5 drachms.
Benzoin	2 ounces.

Cachou à l'Orange.

Powdered catechu . .	4	ounces.
" sugar . . .	24	"

Mix by moistening with a little neroli and oil of Portugal. Dilute with mucilage, stir until well mixed, and divide in grains and dry.

Cachou à la Rose.

Powdered catechu . .	4	ounces.
Mucilage	4	"
Powdered sugar . . .	24	"
Oil of rose	½	drachm.

Prepare as the above.

Cachou à la Vanille.

Powdered catechu . .	4	ounces.
" sugar . . .	24	"
Vanilla cut in small pieces .	2	"

Rub the vanilla, in a marble mortar, with a little catechu and sugar; add the powders from time to time, and rub until the vanilla is reduced to powder; then pour in the mucilage, and triturate so as to obtain a homogeneous paste.

Catechu Pastilles of the Codex.

Extract of liquorice . .	3½	ounces.
Water	3½	"

Melt over a water-bath and add—

Powdered catechu	. .	1 ounce.
" gum	. . .	½ "

Evaporate to the consistency of honey and incorporate—

Finely-powdered mastic	.	½ drachm.
" " cascarilla	.	½ "
" " charcoal	.	½ "
" " orris	.	½ "

Leave on the fire, stir briskly, and, when the mass has consistency enough, remove it from the fire and add—

Oil of mint	. . .	½ drachm.
Tincture of musk	. .	½ "
" ambergris	.	½ "

Run on an oiled marble, and spread with a brush. When the paste is cold, rub it with tissue paper moisten it slightly, and cover it with silver leaf. Dry and cut into lozenges.

Yellow Pastils.

Powdered sandal wood	.	1 pound.
Benzoin	. . . . .	1½ "
Tolu	. . . . . .	4 ounces.
Oil of sandal	. . .	3 drachms.
" cassia	. . .	3 "
" cloves	. . .	3 "
Nitrate of potash	. .	1½ ounce.

Mucilage of tragacanth in sufficient quantity to make the whole into a stiff mass.

Incense Powders.

Powdered sandal wood	.	1 pound.
" cascarilla	. .	8 ounces.
" benzoin	. .	8 "
" vitivert	. .	2 "
" nitrate of potash	.	2 "
Musk	. . . . .	¼ drachm.

Pass the whole several times through a fine sieve.

Perfumers' Pastils.

Charcoal	. . . . .	1 pound.
Benzoin	. . . . .	12 ounces.
Tolu	. . . . . .	4 "
Vanilla	. . . . .	4 "
Cloves	. . . . .	4 "
Oil of sandal	. . .	2 drachms.
" neroli	. . . .	2 "
Nitre	. . . . . .	1½ ounce.
Mucilage of tragacanth	.	1½ "

Eau pour Bruler.

Rectified alcohol	. .	1 pint.
Benzoic acid	. . . .	4 drachms.
Oil of thyme	. . . .	1 drachm.
" caraway	. . . .	1 "
" bergamot	. . . .	2 ounces.

Batons Aromatiques Russes (*to perfume apartments*).

Balsam of Peru	. . .	4½ drachms.
" Mecca	. .	4½ "
" Tolu	. . .	20 "
Storax	. . . .	20 "
Benzoin	. . . .	20 "
Powdered cinnamon	. .	20 "
" cascarilla	. .	20 "
" cloves	. .	4½ "
Sugar	. . . . .	20 "
Vanilla	. . . .	10 "
Musk	. . . . .	¼ drachm.
Ambergris	. . . .	¼ "
Amber	. . . .	40 drachms.
Carminated lake	. . .	4½ "
Oil of rose	. . . .	10 drops.

Make into sticks.

SECTION XIII.

FATTY SUBSTANCES USED IN PERFUMERY.

THE fatty substances used in perfumery are of two kinds—the greases, and the fixed oils.

The greases are solid, soft, or concrete, and are found in the meshes of the cellular or adipose tissue of various animals. The greases are insoluble in water, and lighter than that liquid; inflammable when sufficiently heated; when exposed to the air and light, they become rancid by absorbing a large portion of oxygen, and are thus transformed into acid. All greases are colorless when pure; in an impure state they differ in color—some are white, as those of pork, sheep, calf, etc.; some are yellow, as butter, etc. Greases differ also in odor, consistency, and fusibility; the odor is very weak in tallow and lard, strong and disagreeable in the bear and goat. Generally, greases from carnivorous animals have not much consistency, whilst those from herbivorous animals are more solid. Their solubility is variable, either as they are obtained from animals of different species, or from different parts of the same animal, or of animals of the same species which have suddenly died or have been affected by long-continued disease. The fusibility of greases varies from 80° to 140°, depending upon their immediate composition.

Until 1831, fatty substances were considered as pure immediate principles, differing from each other only in their physical properties; about that time, MM. Chevreul and Braconnot ascertained that fatty substances are mixtures of several peculiar principles, amongst which *margarin*, *stearin*, and *olein* are the most remarkable.

Greases, especially lard and mutton suet, melted with olive oil, are the bases of many pomades, cosmetics, soaps, etc.

Animal greases by time become rancid, and give to the products into the composition of which they enter irritating and sometimes toxical properties.

The greases thus changed, treated by boiling alcohol, leave, after evaporation, a brown residuum having a nauseous taste. This residuum has sometimes poisoned animals.

Greases are adulterated with feculæ, cooked potatoes, kaolin, powdered chalk, etc. All these impurities may be detected by ether, which dissolves only the pure grease. By boiling the suspected grease in ten times its weight of water, all the impurities are precipitated, whilst it floats on the surface.

The oils are liquid, unctuous, and inflammable,

and are extracted from many animal, vegetable, and mineral substances. They are distinguished as fixed and volatile oils.

Fixed oils are similar to liquefied greases; they are inflammable when heated in contact with fire, are not soluble in water, alcohol, and ether, and are transformed into soaps by the action of alkalies. Nearly all vegetable oils are extracted from seeds or stones of fruits, except olive oil, which is obtained from the fruit. Some are extracted for culinary purposes, some for lighting, and others for the manufacture of soaps and other industrial uses, etc.

Animal oils, such as those from fishes, neat's foot, whale, etc., are exclusively employed in industry by certain trades. Mineral oils, properly speaking, are nothing but bitumen. They are extracted from coal, petroleum, asphaltum, etc. They are obtained by distillation. Fixed vegetable oils are generally prepared by pressure. The pulp of the fruits, or the stones, are at first macerated over naked fire or steam; then submitted to the action of the press. But the oils prepared by the cold method are always of the better quality.

The fixed oils are also distinguished as *siccatives* and *non siccative* or *fatty oils.*

Siccative oil, as linseed, hempseed, etc., have the property of thickening by degrees when in contact with the air, and are transformed into a kind of transparent membrane. The fatty oils do not become resinous by the contact of the air.

Fatty oils are insoluble in water, soluble in alcohol and ether, and composed of one or more organic acids in combination with glycerin. They are distinguished from volatile oils by a series of peculiar properties. They may be saponified by alkalies. In this reaction the alkali (potash, soda, ammonia, lime, etc.) is substituted for the glycerin, and combines with the fatty acid, which is most usually stearic, margaric, or oleic. The oleate of glycerin predominates in the fatty oils, while fatty bodies, solid at the ordinary temperature, are richer in the stearate and margarate. Fatty oils, subjected to the action of heat, experience a characteristic decomposition. They generally begin to boil at a temperature between 572° and 752°. They disengage a volatile gas, which has a strongly irritating action on the respiratory organs; at the same time they are discolored and become thick. The siccative (drying) oils then lose their property of being soluble in alcohol and ether, and alter more rapidly when in contact with the air. By cooling they often deposit a certain quantity of their crystallizable acid. At a temperature above that of melted lead, oils are rapidly decomposed; inflammable gas, carbonic acid, and acrolein are disengaged. The products of the decomposition vary according to the duration of the operation. Oleic acid furnishes sebacic acid, and acrolein is formed at the expense of the glycerin. The inflammable products are different forms of carburetted hydrogen.

Fixed oils are often adulterated by being mixed with oils of a cheaper quality or by common animal fats. To detect the adulteration of oils, M. Boudet has proposed a process founded on the different colors produced by the action of hyponitric acid on the different oils, and also the time they take to solidify. All oils not siccative solidify under the influence of this acid. M. Boudet has presented the following table of the reaction of hyponitric acid on different oils:—

Oils.	Coloration they take, immediately after their mixture with the reagent.	Number of minutes before the solidification.	Ratio of time, that of olive oil being 10.
		Minutes.	Minutes.
Olive . . .	Bluish-green	73	10.
Sweet almonds . .	Dirty white	160	22.2
Bitter almonds . .	Dark green	160	22.2
Hazelnut . . .	Bluish-green	103	14.0
Cashewnut . .	Sulphur yellow	43	6.0
Castor . . .	Golden yellow	603	82.6
Colza . . .	Brownish-yellow	2400	328.0
Black poppy . .	Slightly yellow		
Beech . . .	Pink		
Hazelnut . . .	Pink		

The experiments were made at a temperature of 62°.6 on 1¼ drachm of each oil, and with 1 grain of a mixture of three parts nitric acid at 35° B., and one part hyponitric acid.

The principal oils used in perfumery are the hazelnut oil, the oil of behn, the oils of sweet and bitter almonds, etc.

CHAPTER XXVII.

OILS—GREASES—WAX.

Olive Oil

Is extracted from the fruit of the European olive tree (*olea Europea*).

It is very fluid, unctuous, transparent, slightly odoriferous when new, but becomes rancid in time. Sometimes it has a greenish-yellow color, sometimes pale yellow, sometimes colorless. Its taste is sweet and agreeable. Its density varies according to the temperature.

At 53°.6	it is	0.9192
At 122°	"	0.8932
At 201°.2	"	0.8625

It may be mixed with gum water. A few degrees above the freezing point, olive oil becomes nebulous and begins to deposit stearin; at 21°.2 it deposits 0.28 stearine, and leaves 0.72 of olein. It begins to boil at 622°.4, assuming a darker color. Its solubility in alcohol and ether when the oil is fresh, is the same as that of oil of sweet almonds, one thousand drops of alcohol dissolving three drops of oil. According to Braconnot, olive oil is composed of seventy-two parts of olein and twenty-eight of stearin. It is employed in perfumery to prepare cosmetic pastes and pomades, and also to manufacture soaps.

Oil of Behn.

Is extracted by expression from the BEHN, fruit of the *moringa aptera*, now naturalized in the West Indies. It is sweet, nearly colorless, becomes rancid with difficulty, odorless, with an agreeable taste. Its density equals 0.902; at 59° it is thick; in winter it is solid, neutral to test papers. At a low temperature the oil separates in two parts, one solid composed of *stearin* and *margarin*, the other liquid *olein*, which will not freeze. This oil contains four fatty solid acids: the *stearic*, *margaric*, *behnic*, and *moringic*.

This is the finest fat oil which a perfumer could use, on account of the property of not becoming rancid. For making cold cream and all kinds of unguents it is invaluable and without a competitor. It is the best oil to enflower.

Oil of Sweet Almonds

Is extracted by expression from the sweet and bitter almonds, fruits of the *Amygdalus communis.*

According to Barclay, sweet almonds have the following composition:—

A yellowish fatty oil, very sweet .	0.54
Albumen	0.24
Sugar	0.06
Gum	0.03
Outside pellicles	0.05
Fibrous parts	0.05
Acetic acid	traces.
	0.97

According to Vogel, bitter almonds contain—

Fat oil	26
Uncrystallized sugar . . .	0.5
Gum	3.0
Ligneous fibre	5.0
Pericarp	8.5
Caseous matter	"
Prussic acid . .	undetermined quantity.

The oil of sweet almonds is of a light yellow color, with an agreeable taste, without odor, and very fluid. At 59° its density is from 0.917 to 0.920.

At 14° it gives 0.24 stearine fusible at 42°.8, and 0.76 oleine.

It completely solidifies at —13°.

Good sweet almond oil ought not to have any smell of rancidity or prussic acid. It is very soluble in ether; alcohol dissolves only one twenty-fourth of its weight.

It is largely employed in perfumes.

Palm Oil

Is extracted from the fruit of the *Elæis guineensis*, or *Avoira elæis*, of the family of palm-trees.

Commercial palm oil is solid, of an orange-yellow color, with a buttery consistency. Its taste is sweet and perfumed, its odor similar to that of orris-root or violet.

Recently made, it melts at 80°.6; but the melting point rises to 88°, and even 100°, by age.

It is insoluble in water, soluble in cold alcohol, more soluble in warm alcohol, but is partially precipitated on cooling. Soluble in all proportions in ether.

It is easily saponified, and gives a yellow soap. According to M. Henry, it is composed of 31 parts of stearine and 69 of oleine, a coloring principle combined with oleine, and a volatile odoriferous principle.

It is used to make soaps. Sometimes the oil is bleached, for the purpose of making white soaps. In the next chapter we shall describe the process employed for bleaching it.

Coco Oil.

Extracted by expression or by fusion from the kernel of the fruit of some coco trees (*Cocos nucifera*, *Elæis butyracea*). The nut of the coco contains—

	Per cent.
Oil	71.488
Zimon	7.665
Mucilage	3.588
Cryst. glycin	1.595
Yellow coloring principle	0.325
Ligneous fibre	14.950
Loss	0.392

The oil is white, and in warm climates is as fluid and limpid as water; it solidifies between 60° and 64°.4. In this state it melts at 68°. When fresh its odor and taste are sweet and agreeable. It becomes rancid very quickly.

It contains two principles, one solid and the other liquid. The solid principle is a peculiar acid, *coccinic*, combined with glycerine.

Used in the manufacture of toilet soaps; sometimes also in the preparation of pomades.

Oil and Butter of Nutmegs

Are extracted from the nutmeg, fruit of the *Myristica aromatica, Myristica officinalis, Myristica moschata.*

The nutmeg contains two oils, one volatile, the other fixed and concrete; the first is whitish-yellow, lighter than water, with an acrid taste and a strong odor of nutmeg; the second is white, without taste and odor when pure.

The butter of nutmeg has a pale yellow color; its taste and odor are strong and sweet. It is composed of—

Concrete oil similar to myristin .	43.07
Butyrous yellow oil . . .	58.08
Volatile oil	4.85

Distilled, it furnishes about $\frac{1}{18}$ of its weight of volatile oil.

Used in compound perfumes.

Butter of Cacao

Is obtained from the roasted seeds of the cacao-tree, *Theobroma cacao.*

Pure and recently prepared, its color is yellowish, but becomes white by age. Its odor and taste are sweet. It can be kept a long time without turning rancid. Soluble in warm alcohol, very soluble in ether and spirit of turpentine.

When pure, it melts at 84°.2, and solidifies at 73°.4. Its density = 0.91.

It is composed of a substance fusible at 84°.2, in which stearine is combined with oleine.

Is used sometimes in pomades and cosmetic creams.

Tallow

Is the melted grease of beef, mutton, veal, etc. These three are most used in perfumery.

Beef tallow is pinkish-white, and hard; it may be kept in a cool place without moulding. When melted, it is grayish-white, hard, and opalescent. After being melted, it begins to solidify at 98°.6;

its temperature then rises to 102°.2. It requires 40 parts of alcohol to dissolve it.

Veal tallow, when crude, is pinkish-white, melts easily between the fingers, is very soft, and opalescent. After melting, it becomes milk-white, nacreous, and soft. It decomposes very easily, and much faster than sheep tallow.

Sheep tallow has the external appearance of beef tallow. It is white-pinkish, hard, and opalescent in thin cakes. It moulds very easily. When melted, it is milky-white, and has a nacreous appearance.

Exposed for some time to the air, it acquires a peculiar odor.

When melted, it begins sometimes to solidify at 98°.6, and the temperature rises to 102°.2; sometimes it begins to solidify at 104°, and the temperature rises to 105°.8. It requires 44 parts of boiling alcohol to dissolve one part of sheep tallow.

In the next chapter we shall give the process for purifying these greases.

Lard

Is extracted from the adipose tissue overlying the kidneys and intestines of the hog. It is white or slightly yellowish, soft at the ordinary temperature, and nearly odorless. Its fusibility is variable between 47° and 56°.

Its density at 59° is 0.938. When pressed, it

gives 0.62 of its weight of a colorless oleine. Exposed to the air for some time, it becomes yellow and rancid, and acquires a strong odor. It contains 38 per cent. of stearine and 62 of oleine.

One hundred parts of lard give by saponification 9 of glycerine and 94.65 of fatty acids which solidify at 125°.6. Lard dissolves in 36 parts of boiling alcohol.

Spermaceti.

This fatty material exists in solution in the oil found in the head of some species of cachalots, principally the *Physeter macrocephalus.*

Spermaceti is semitransparent, soft, producing under the fingers the same sensation as hard soap. It is brittle, insipid, odorless, fusible at 113°. Its density at 59° = 0.943. It cannot be saponified.

Exposed to the air, it becomes yellow and acid, and acquires a rancid odor. Insoluble in water, more soluble in warm than in cold alcohol, ether, fixed and volatile oils. 100 parts of boiling alcohol dissolve 3.5 of spermaceti, of which 0.9 deposit by cooling.

Spermaceti is found in the market in the form of white, half-transparent, brittle cakes, with a crystalline and lamelloid fracture.

In perfumery it enters into the composition of cold cream, pomades, pastes, etc. It is considered as one of the best constituents of cosmetics.

Wax

Is a substance secreted by bees, an insect belonging to the family of the *Melliferes.*

There are two kinds, *yellow wax* and *white wax.* The latter being the most used, we shall examine its properties.

It is white, slightly diaphanous, without taste, odorless, hard and brittle at 32°. Malleable at 86°, it becomes soft when heated, and at 149° is entirely liquid. Is decomposed by boiling.

Insoluble in water, partially soluble in alcohol, soluble in ether, the fixed and essential oils. Its density = 0.960. It is inflammable, and burns without residuum, giving a very bright flame. Is employed in the composition of cerates, cold creams, cosmetics, and some pomades.

Paraffine

Is a solid, wax-like, inodorous substance, obtained at first by low distillation of mineral boghead, peat, but more recently was found very abundantly in petroleum. It is an article that will find several uses in perfumery as a substitute for wax and spermaceti. It will be a valuable adjunct in the manufacture of powders which have to be exported to hot climates. It is completely neutral, and has great stability, alkalies and concentrated acids having no action upon it. Its specific gravity = 0.37. At 112° it melts into a colorless oil, but the heat may be gradually increased to 698° without producing any decomposition. It is soluble in spirit of turpentine and naphtha. Boiling ether dissolves it largely, but deposits it by cooling. Boiling absolute alcohol dissolves from three to four per cent., but drops it on cooling. Its composition is—

Carbon	85.22
Hydrogen	14.78

CHAPTER XXVIII.

EPURATION AND PREPARATION OF GREASES FOR POMADE BODIES.

Purification of Lard.

TAKE 28 pounds of perfectly fresh lard; place it in a well-glazed vessel that can be submitted to the heat of a boiling salt-water bath, or of steam under a slight pressure. When the lard is melted, add to it one ounce of powdered alum and two ounces of table salt. Maintain the heat for some time—in fact, till a scum rises, consisting in a great measure of coagulated proteine compounds, membrane, etc., which must be skimmed off. When the liquid grease appears of a uniform nature, it is allowed to cool.

The lard is now to be washed. This is done in small quantities at a time, and is a work of much labor; which, however, is amply repaid by the result. About one pound of the grease is placed on a slate slab, a little on the incline, a supply of good water being set to trickle over it. The surface of the grease is then constantly renewed by an operative working a muller over it, precisely as a color-maker grinds paints in oil. In this way the water removes any traces of alum or soap; also the last traces of nitrogeneous matter. Finally, the grease, when the whole is washed in this way, is remelted, the heat being maintained sufficiently to throw off any adhering water. When cold, the operation is finished.

Purification of Beef and Mutton Suet.

Take 100 pounds of perfectly fresh suet; cut it into small pieces, and pound it well in a mortar. When it is well crushed wash it with water repeatedly—so long, in fact, as the water is not as clear after withdrawing the grease as before it was put in. The grease has now to be melted over a slow fire, adding thereto about three ounces of powdered alum and a handful of kitchen salt. Let the grease boil, but allow it to bubble for a few seconds only; then strain the grease through fine linen into a deep pan, and allow it to stand, to clear itself from all impurities, for about two hours. The clear grease is again to be put into the pan, over a bright fire, adding thereto about three or four quarts of rose water, and about five ounces of powdered gum benzoin. It is allowed to heat gently, and all scum that rises is to be removed until it ceases to be produced. Finally, the grease is put into deep pans, and, when cold, taken carefully off the sedimentary water. It is then fit for use, and may be kept for an indefinite period without change or turning rancid.

The object of the benzoin is to prevent the grease becoming rancid.

Bleaching of Palm Oil.

This operation is rarely resorted to on account of the oil losing some of its fine odor.

The oil is melted in a kettle over a water bath, and for every 100 pounds of oil, 10 pounds of powdered peroxide of manganese are thrown in. Stir the mass to incorporate well, and, after ten or fifteen minutes, pour into it 4 pounds of sulphuric acid. Increase the heat until ebullition commences, stirring from time to time; then let it cool. The oil has a greenish shade, and rises to the surface of the water. Separate the oil, expose it to the air, and it becomes white in a short time. In England they employ a more simple process; it consists in exposing the oil to the action of the air at a temperature of 212°. In a few days the oil is bleached, and can be used to manufacture white soaps.

SECTION XIV.

POMADES—CREAM CERATES—COLD CREAMS—SERKIS, ETC.

SOFT and unctuous compounds, prepared with wax or grease of some animals, with which other substances are mixed according to their uses. At Grasse they are obtained by or without infusion. Those made by the first method are the pomades of rose, orange flower, and acacia; the others are the pomades of jasmine, tuberose, jonquil, narcisse, violet, etc. In Paris they generally make pomades by composition; the oils used are ordinarily those of bergamot, lemon, etc. The good quality of a pomade depends on the purity and freshness of the substances which compose it, and the mode of preparation. If the oils and greases are old, or if too much heated, the pomade becomes bad; then, to avoid loss, they are colored, and their perfume changed.

Pomades prepared cold, and beaten in a mortar, are the best, and the least susceptible of rancidity.

CHAPTER XXIX.

POMADES.

Pommade à la Rose—By Infusion.

TAKE one pound of grease, prepared as we have described in the preceding chapter; introduce it into a kettle with one pound of fresh rose leaves, perfectly free from dampness. Mix them well, and melt over a water bath; keep melted one day, stirring as often as possible. Pass the grease through a fine sieve; press the leaves so as to extract the grease and odoriferous principle they contain. Repeat the operation with one pound of fresh leaves four or five times, observing the same precautions. The more frequently this is repeated the better the pomade. When the pomade is passed for the last time, introduce into the jar, and mix with it 1½ drachm of oil of geranium, and stir well with a spatula, so as to incorporate the oil. Allow the pomade to cool; keep it in porcelain jars, sheltered from light and dust.

This mode of preparation may be applied to all the pomades manufactured with flowers.

Pommade à la Rose—By Composition.

Prepared grease	. .	1 pound.
Spermaceti	. . .	2 ounces.
Oil of sweet almonds	. .	3 "
" roses	. . .	¼ drachm.
" geranium	. . .	¼ "

Melt together the grease, oil, and spermaceti over a water bath. During the fusion stir with a spatula; when melted, pour the mass into a marble mortar; wait until it begins to solidify; then, with the pestle, triturate until a homogeneous white pomade is obtained. Pour in the oils, and triturate a long time to incorporate them. A few drachms of alcoholate of roses may be added. If a rose color is wanted, heat the three ounces of oil with half a drachm of alkanet, and pass through a sieve; the oil has then the required color.

Pommade au Jasmin.

Prepared grease	. .	2 pounds.
Storax	. . . .	1 ounce.
Benzoin	. . . .	1 "

Melt over a water bath, and infuse one day.

Next day melt again; pass through a fine sieve; place over a water bath, and introduce into the mass—

Pomade with orange flower	10 ounces.
" " cassia	5 "

When the mass begins to melt, add—

Jasmine flowers . . . 24 ounces.

Stir some time with a spatula; take from the fire, and let it infuse twenty-four hours. After this time, melt over a water bath; strain, press, and add a few drops of oils of amber and musk. Stir well, and put in small porcelain jars.

Pommade à la Fleur d'Orange.

Prepared grease . .	1 pound.
Fresh orange flowers . .	8 ounces.

Operate in the same manner as for the rose, and at the end of the operation add—

Oil of bergamot . . . ½ drachm.

Pommade à la Violette.

Prepared grease . .	1 pound.
Cassia pomade . . .	8 ounces.
Jasmine " . . .	8 "

Melt, and add—

Violet flowers . . . 1 pound.

Operate as for the roses.

Pommade à la Tubereuse.

Prepared grease . . .	1 pound.
Storax	4 ounces.

Melt, and incorporate the storax; then add—

Orange-flower pomade .	4 ounces.
Jasmine " " . .	4 "

Triturate quickly, to effect the mixture; then add—

Tuberose flowers . . 4 ounces.

Continue the operation as for the rose.

Pommade à la Cassie.

Prepared grease . . .	2 pounds.
Storax	4 ounces.
Benzoin	4 "

Melt, strain, and add—

Cassia flowers . . . 1 pound.

Let it infuse twenty-four hours. After this time, stir the grease well with the flowers, melt a third time, and during the fusion add—

Jasmine pomade . . 5 ounces.

The whole being melted, strain and press in the same manner as for the rose.

The pomades with *reseda, jonquil, hyacinth, lilac, heliotrope, syringa,* etc., are all prepared in the same manner.

Pommade à la Vanille.

Prepared grease . . .	1 pound.
Storax	1 ounce.
Benzoin	1 "

Melt, digest three days; melt again, pass through a sieve, and add—

Vanilla cut in small pieces . 1 ounce.

Mix the vanilla well with the grease, macerate ten days, being careful to stir several times a day. After this time, melt over a water bath, pass through a sieve, and press well the residuum. When the mass begins to solidify, add—

Oil of bergamot	. . .	¼ drachm.
" cloves	. . .	¼ "
Tincture of vanilla	. .	½ "
" balsam of Peru		¼ "
" benzoin	. .	½ "

Beat well, to incorporate the perfumes.

Pommade au Bouquet.

Melt over a water bath—

Orange-flower pomade	.	3½ ounces.
Tuberose	. . . .	3½ "
Jonquil	. . . .	3½ "
Cassia	. . . .	3½ "

When melted, add—

Jasmine pomade	. .	1 pound.

Stir well, and, when the mass begins to solidify, add—

Oil of bergamot	. . .	1 drachm.
" cloves	. . .	2 drachms.
" white thyme	. .	8 grains.

Stir and beat, to incorporate.

Pommade aux Millefleurs

Is prepared as the above, but the following are added:—

Oil of Portugal	. . .	1 drachm.
" lavender	. . .	½ "
" vervain	. . .	¼ "

Pommade Ambrée et Musquée.

Musk	. . . .	¼ drachm.
Ambergris	. . . .	½ "
Prepared grease	. . .	1 pound.

Triturate the musk and ambergris in a mortar with a little alcohol; take two ounces of the grease and triturate it with the ambergris and musk; put all the grease in a kettle, and melt it over a water bath; when just melted, take it off, and let it digest ten days. After this time, melt again, and add—

Vanilla pomade	. . .	5 ounces.
Jasmine "	. . . .	5 "
Tuberose "	. . . .	3½ "

Strain, and introduce into porcelain jars.

Pommade à la Moelle de Bœuf.

Beef marrow	. . .	12 ounces.
Prepared grease	. . .	8 "
Olive oil	. . . .	1 ounce.
White wax	. . .	2 ounces.
Juice of a lemon.		

Melt and incorporate well.

Pommade Philocome.

Beef marrow . . .	1 ounce.
Oil of sweet almonds . .	2 drachms.
Extract of cinchona . .	½ drachm.
Balsam of Peru . . .	20 drops.
Oil of bergamot . . .	8 "

Pommade Transparente.

Spermaceti	2 ounces.
Castor oil	5 "
Alcohol	5 "
Oil of bergamot . . .	½ drachm.
" Portugal . . .	½ "

Melt together the spermaceti and castor oil, pour in the alcohol by degrees, stop the heat, and add the oils. Stir well, to incorporate, and pour into glass jars.

CHAPTER XXX.

POMADES WITH ESSENTIAL OILS.

POMADES are also manufactured without macerating the flowers in the grease; they are made with greases and essential oils. They are as good as the above, and have the advantage of keeping longer; greases heated several times, soon become rancid. We give as specimens the following pomades, which can be prepared according to the taste.

White Pomade.

Purified veal grease[1] . .	14 ounces.
Spermaceti . . .	4 "
White wax . . .	1 ounce.
Behn or almond oil . .	8 ounces.

Melt over a water bath, pour into a mortar, triturate well until a homogeneous paste is obtained, then add—

Oil of bitter almonds .	½ drachm.
" geranium . .	2½ drachms.
" bergamot . .	4 "
Tincture of musk . .	¼ drachm.

Beat until perfectly incorporated.

[1] For its purification, see chapter *New Products*.

Prepare in the same manner all the pomades with essential oils.

Pomade in Sticks.

This pomade, which is used to smooth the hair, ought to present a hard body which will retain its form under pressure. The substances which enter into its composition are—

Purified beef tallow . .	10 ounces.
Wax	2 "

Melt over a water bath, and when the mass begins to cool, aromatize according to taste; stir well, and run into moulds.

This pomade is colored in the following manner:—

Black, with powdered charcoal or ivory black.
Yellow, with carbonate of iron or annotto.
Rose, with alkanet, lake, or cochineal.
Green, with chlorophyl, etc.

CHAPTER XXXI.

PERFUMED HAIR OILS.

Antique Oil.

Behn oil	1 pound.
Oil of bergamot . .	4 drachms.
Tincture of ambergris .	2½ "

Huile des Celèbes.

Pure olive oil . . .	1 pound.
Yellow sandal . . .	1 ounce.
Cinnamon . . .	4 drachms.

Digest the sandal and cinnamon in the oil, strain and add—

Oil of Portugal . . .	1 drachm.

Oil of Macassar.

Oil of sunflower seeds .	3 ounces.
Goose fat	1 ounce.
Butter of Cacao . . .	2 drachms.
Oil of eggs . . .	2 "
Storax	2 "
Neroli	1 drachm.
Oil of thyme . . .	½ "
Balsam of Peru . . .	8 drops.
Oil of roses . . .	1 drop.

Mix the whole, macerate one night, and filter.

CHAPTER XXXII.

ANTICALVITIC AND REGENERATIVE POMADES.

Pomade to Prevent Baldness (*Bouchardat*).

Lard	1 ounce.
Lemon juice . . .	1½ drachm.
Tincture of Spanish flies .	½ "

Pomade for Alopecia (*Steege*).

Butter of cacao . . .	1⅓ ounces.
Olive oil	⅔ ounce.
Quinia	6 drops.
Tannin	9 "
Aromatic tincture . .	15 "

Regenerative Pomade.

Lard	5 ounces.
Carbonate of soda . .	1 ounce.
Tartar emetic . . .	½ drachm.
Medicated soap . . .	1 ounce.

Pomade with Butternut Leaves.

Prepared grease . . .	1 pound.
Fresh butternut leaves .	8 ounces.
Tincture of parsley seeds .	2 drachms.
Oil of lavender . . .	½ drachm.
" marjoram . . .	½ "
" cloves . . .	1 "

Triturate the leaves in a mortar, and, when mashed, throw them on the grease; melt over a water bath. When melted, check the heat, and digest for three days. Then melt, pass through a sieve, pour into it the tincture of parsley, and heat well; add the oils, and stir until perfectly incorporated.

Anticalvitic Powder.

Powdered parsley seeds .	2 ounces.
Cinchona	4 drachms.
Catechu	2½ "

Mix, and pass through a sieve.

Pomade for Baldness.

Prepared grease . . .	1 pound.
Alcoholic extract of cinchona	1 ounce.
Tannin	½ drachm.
Tar	¼ "

Triturate in a mortar the tar and cinchona; add the tannin, with a little alcohol and soap, to dissolve it better; then put in the grease, and triturate until well mixed. Perfume with a few drops of oil of cloves and cinnamon.

CHAPTER XXXIII.

COSMETIC POMADES FOR THE SKIN.

Cold Cream.

Spermaceti	. . .	2½ ounces.
White wax	. . .	1 ounce.
Oil of sweet almonds	. .	10 ounces.

Melt over a water bath, and pour into a mortar. Triturate and beat until a white cream free from grains is obtained, adding by degrees—

Triple rose water	. .	2 ounces.

Towards the end of the operation, perfume with—

Oil of rose	. . .	10 drops.
Tincture of benzoin	. .	5 "
" ambergris	.	2 "

Beat again. The more it is beaten the whiter and better it will be.

Pommade aux Concombres.

Purified grease	. . .	1 pound.
Spermaceti	. . .	5 ounces.
White wax	. . .	1 ounce.
Oil of behn	. . .	5 ounces.

Melt over a water bath, and add—

Cucumber juice . . .	10 ounces.

Heat three or four hours, press, and allow it to cool. Separate from the aqueous part, melt again, press a second time; let it cool, to separate the water which is left. Throw the pomade into a marble mortar, and beat it two hours, adding a little more water and glycerine.

Pommade à la Sultane.

Spermaceti . . .	2 ounces.
White wax . . .	1 ounce.
Oil of almonds . . .	4 ounces.
Rose water . . .	1 ounce.
Mecca balsam . . .	4 drachms.

Melt together over a water bath the wax, spermaceti, and oil. Pour into a marble mortar, and beat until homogeneous. Lastly, add—beating all the time—the balsam and rose water.

Crême du Cattay.

Turpentine . . .	½ drachm.
Spermaceti . . .	2 drachms.
White wax . . .	1 drachm.
White oxide of zinc . .	1 "
Oil of almonds . . .	4 ounces.
Rose water . . .	6 "
Oil of roses . . .	¼ drachm.

Melt over a water bath, triturate with the rose water, and add the oxide of zinc.

Crême du Liban.

Oil of behn . . .	8 ounces.
" poppy . . .	2 "
White wax . . .	½ ounce.
Spermaceti . . .	1 "
Benzoic acid . . .	1 "
Almond milk . . .	16 ounces.
White of bismuth . .	8 "
Talc	4 "
Balsam of Peru . . .	¼ drachm.
Oil of rose . . .	1 grain.

Make a pomade.

Pommade Rosat.

Prepared grease . . .	2 ounces.
Oil of sweet almonds . .	1 ounce.
White wax . . .	1½ "
Alkanet	¼ drachm.

Melt over a water bath; pass through a sieve; pour into a mortar, and triturate until homogeneoous. Then add—

Oil of roses . . .	12 drops.

Triturate until incorporated.

Instead of alkanet, carmin may be used.

Camphorated Pomade.

Prepared grease . . .	8 ounces.
Spermaceti . . .	2 "
White wax . . .	1 ounce.
Oil of sweet almonds . .	8 ounces.

Melt over a water bath; run into a marble mortar; let it cool, and when nearly solidified, triturate until homogeneous. Then add—

Camphor	4 drachms.

The camphor must be previously powdered by triturating with a few drops of alcohol. Incorporate it in the pomade.

Pommade d'Hebé, for wrinkles.

Incorporate together—

Juice of tubers of white lily	2 ounces.
Honey	4 drachms.
White wax . . .	1 ounce.
Rose water . . .	3 drachms.

Melt the wax over a water bath; then add the other substances; stir until well incorporated.

Pommade de Beauté, for chapped skin.

Melt together over a water bath—

White wax . . .	1½ drachm.
Spermaceti . . .	2 drachms.
Oil of sweet almonds . .	4 "
Olive oil	4 "
Poppy oil	4 "

Beat well, and introduce—

Liquid balsam of Peru .	4 drops.

Pomade with Butter of Cacao.

Prepared grease . .	8 ounces.
Almond oil . . .	5 "
Butter of cacao	10 "

Melt; pour into a mortar; triturate well, and perfume with essence of vanilla.

Astringent Pomade.

Nutgalls	1 ounce.
Cypress nut . . .	1 "
Pomegranate bark . .	1 "
Sumach	1 "
Oil of myrtle . . .	4 ounces.
Pommade rosat . . .	20 "

Boil the vegetable substances in one pint of water. Continue the ebullition until reduced to four ounces. Filter, and press; mix with the pomade, and cool; triturate in a mortar until well incorporated. Perfume according to taste.

Another.

Pommade rosat . . .	1 pound.
Tannin	1 drachm.
Pure sulphate of zinc . .	¼ drachm.

Dissolve the sulphate of zinc and tannin in a little rose water; pour into a mortar on the pomade, and triturate until well incorporated.

Pomade with Tar.

Prepared grease . . .	1 ounce.
Tar	½ drachm.

Add a little camphor.

Sulphuretted Pomade.

Sublimed sulphur, washed with rose water . .	4 ounces.
Cold cream . . .	1 ounce.

Triturate in a mortar until well mixed, and add—

Cherry-laurel water . .	1 ounce.

Triturate again.

Pomade to paste Wigs.

Isinglass	1 ounce.
Water	8 ounces.

Melt, and add—

Alcohol	8 ounces.
Tincture of benzoin . .	2 "
Turpentine . . .	2 ".

Place over a water bath, and mix.

SECTION XV.

DEPILATORIES.

SUBSTANCES more or less caustic, generally dangerous, used for the purpose of destroying hairs on the skin. Quicklime and sulphide of arsenic form the basis of nearly all of them. A. Paré advises to inclose in a rag equal parts of these two substances, and after dipping them in water to rub the part to be depilated. The *rusma* of the Turks, which appears to be the best, is prepared with 2 ounces of lime, ½ ounce sulphide of arsenic, which are boiled in one pound of an alkaline lye, until by dipping a quill into the mixture the liquid is strong enough to separate the feathers. It is spread on the part, and, a few seconds after, a simple sponging with warm water will remove all the hairs. Sometimes it is sufficient to prepare, in the same proportions, a powder, which is afterwards diluted with a little water to apply in the form of paste. This mixture is rendered less corrosive by incorporating into it rye flour, starch, or paste of sweet almonds. Sulphide of barium moistened with a little water, the ointment of quicklime of Minsicht, and the trochists of arsenic have also been used; but all of these articles must be employed very carefully, especially when arsenic enters into their composition, for a prolonged application will produce a real poisoning by the absorption of a certain quantity of the arsenic. They have also this other inconvenience—that they corrode the skin. Whatever are the effects of these dangerous cosmetics, they do not prevent the hairs from growing again, and consequently they must be frequently used.

CHAPTER XXXIV.

FORMULÆ FOR DEPILATORIES.

Depilatory Powder of the Perfumers.

Powdered quicklime . .	1 ounce.
" orris root . .	2 ounces.
Sulphide of arsenic . .	1 drachm.

Mix and pass through a fine sieve. To use it, mix some of the powder with water and apply to the hairy part; a few seconds after, rub and the hair will fall off.

Another.

Quicklime	4 drachms.
Sulphide of arsenic . .	¼ drachm.
Starch	2½ drachms.

Mix, pass through a sieve, and keep in well-corked bottles.

Turkish Depilatory.

Quicklime	2 ounces.
Sulphide of arsenic . .	½ ounce.

Boil the whole in 2 pounds of an alkaline lye. This preparation is very dangerous.

Another.

Mercury	2 ounces.
Powdered sulphide of arsenic	1 ounce.
" litharge . .	1 "
" starch . . .	1 "

Rub well together until the mercury is extinct, and pass through a silk sieve and make a paste with soap-water.

Another.

Powdered orris-root . .	3 ounces.
Quicklime	8 "

Another.

Quicklime	1 ounce.
Nitre	1 drachm.
Soap-makers' lye . .	4 ounces.
Sulphide of arsenic . .	3 drachms.

Evaporate to a convenient consistency.

Another.

Quicklime	1 ounce.
Powdered gum . . .	2 ounces.
Sulphide of arsenic . .	1 drachm.

Martin's Depilatory with Sulphuretted Sulphide of Calcium.

Sulphuretted sulphide of calcium	1 ounce.

Apply a light coating on the part to be depilated; after eight or ten minutes wash with water, and the skin is perfectly deprived of hair.

Depilatory with Sulphydrate of Soda.

Powdered quicklime . .	8 ounces.
Starch	12 "
Sulphydrate of soda . .	3½ "
Filtered water . . .	16 "

Dissolve the sulphydrate in water, introduce the lime and starch in a marble mortar, and triturate, adding the sulphydrate little by little; grind until a homogeneous paste is obtained. Keep in blue ground-stoppered bottles.

This depilatory is the best, the most efficacious, and the least dangerous. It must be kept out of the light.

SECTION XVI.

WHITES AND REDS.

PERFUMERY, which is so fecund in odoriferous products, has been unable yet to manufacture harmless whites. Generally the whites it produces are more or less dangerous to the health. Indeed, salts of lead, bismuth, baryta, or zinc, are always the basis of these whites, and it would be a great improvement to produce a white as fine as those already in use, yet free from all those noxious properties.

It is not the same for the reds; perfumery uses several kinds which all belong to the vegetable kingdom, such as the carthamine, garancine, carmine, geranium, etc., all of which are perfectly harmless.

CHAPTER XXXV.

WHITES.

BISMUTH — WHITES OF BISMUTH — CERUSE OR WHITES OF LEAD—WHITE OF ZINC—WHITE OF TALC—WHITE OF BARYTA.

Bismuth.

A METAL of a reddish-white color, very brittle, easy to powder, of a lamellous texture. Its specific gravity equals 9.83. It melts at 399°.2, and by cooling crystallizes in cubes disposed in such a manner that they form a quadrangular pyramid.

Its nitric solution is used to make a sympathetic ink, nearly colorless by itself, but which becomes immediately black by contact with sulphuretted hydrogen; this solution is used to prepare pearl white.

The perfumer ought to purchase the metal in well-defined crystals, so as to have it perfectly free from arsenic. Its use is dangerous.

Pearl White in Trochists.

Pure bismuth	1 pound.
Nitric acid	6 pounds.

Reduce the bismuth to a coarse powder, and introduce it into a porcelain dish with the nitric acid; and when the reaction has ceased, heat it gently until all the metal is dissolved; evaporate the solution to two-thirds, and pour it slowly into fifty times its volume of water. A white substance is precipitated, which is the *subnitrate of bismuth,* or white of pearl. Wash this white with water until it is free from acid; collect it on a cotton cloth, let it drain, and dry it with a gentle heat in a dark room.

Liquid Pearl White.

Subnitrate of bismuth .	1 pound.
Distilled water . . .	3 pounds.

Rub the subnitrate in a marble mortar, add the water little by little, and, when the mass is well mixed, introduce it into bottles of green glass.

Unctuous White in Pomade.

Subnitrate of bismuth .	1 ounce.
Cold cream . . .	2 ounces.

Rub in a mortar until a homogeneous paste is obtained.

Ceruse,

also called *subcarbonate of lead,* is a combination of carbonic acid and oxide of lead. It is white, friable, insipid, and insoluble in water. When pure, it completely dissolves in nitric acid. Ceruse is sold in the form of conical cakes weighing from two to four pounds. It is often mixed with other white substances of less value, such as sulphates of lead and baryta, chalk, plaster, etc.

Ceruse is extensively used in the arts. Perfumers employ it in the composition of some whites. It is one of the most dangerous substances. Its use ought to be rejected. In some cases it has produced poisoning.

Silver White.

This white has sometimes been designated by the name of *snow white.* It is pure carbonate of lead. It may be prepared as a liquid in the same manner as the pearl white.

A preparation is sold which is made in the following manner:—

This white is composed in two bottles. The first contains a filtered solution of acetate of lead; the second, a weak solution of carbonate of soda in rose water.

To use it, fill a wineglass with the liquid of the first bottle; then pour into it two spoonfuls of the liquid of the second bottle. Immediately a very fine white powder of carbonate of lead is precipitated, with which the skin is painted.

Snow White.

Washed oxide of zinc .	1 pound.
Talc	3½ ounces.
Distilled water . . .	3 pounds.

Grind, adding the water little by little. When a homogeneous liquor is obtained, pour into bottles.

White of Talc.

Powdered talc	. . .	1 pound.
Distilled vinegar	. . .	3 pounds.

Pour the talc and the vinegar into a glass balloon, and digest for two weeks, shaking several times a day. Filter and wash the deposit until the water is no longer acid, squeeze it in a white cloth, throw the talc into a marble mortar, and grind it with a little soap water slightly gummy. When the whole is reduced into a paste, fill little porcelain jars, and let it dry.

Baryta White.

Sulphate of baryta	. .	10 ounces.
Oxide of zinc	. . .	1 pound.
Talc	. . . . .	5 ounces.

Make the mixture in a mortar with filtered water, and then pour into vials.

CHAPTER XXXVI.

REDS.

CARTHAMINE—GARANCINE—COCHINEAL—CARMIN—CARMINE—BRESILINE—DIFFERENT FORMS OF RED.

Carthamine

Is the coloring principle of the saffron, *Carthamus tinctorius.* It is obtained in the following manner: wash the flowers of the carthamus with cold water, and continue the washing until the water is no longer colored yellow. Press in a cloth and introduce it into a glass or porcelain vessel, pour over it a solution of carbonate of soda, macerate three hours and strain. Dip into the liquid a skein of cotton and saturate the soda by citric acid. The coloring matter dissolved by the alkali is set free by the acid and combines with the cotton. Wash the skein with cold water and dissolve out the carthamine by a solution of carbonate of soda. The water is colored red; the carthamine is now precipitated by neutralizing the soda with citric acid; let it settle; decant the clear liquor and collect the deposit on a filter. This deposit is the pure red of the carthamus.

Garancine,

Or madder red, is obtained by washing coarsely powdered madder with cold water; after the washing, it is boiled in a concentrated solution of alum. Decant the red liquid and pour into it enough sulphuric acid to acidulate it, and let it rest. A few days after, when a red precipitate has deposited, it is collected. This precipitate is the *garancine* or red principle of madder. Wash it first with cold water, then with hydrochloric acid, so as to dissolve any alumina it may contain. Decant anew and wash with cold water. Filter and dissolve in alcohol. In a few days the alcoholic solution will deposit a crystalline powder of an orange-red color, which being treated by an alkali gives a very fine red.

Cochineal (*Coccus cacti*).

An insect belonging to the family of the *gall insects*, the female of which alone furnishes the rich red color known by the name of *cochineal.* Cochineal is originally from Mexico, in the neighborhood of Guaxaca and Oaxaca.

It is in the *Cactus opuntia* or *nopal* that the cochineal lives and multiplies. The process is very simple: The insects are distributed in groups in nopals planted in rows, with space enough between each to permit a man to pass around them. In a few days the insects begin to multiply with the greatest rapidity. In two months the whole surface of the nopal is entirely covered with cochineal ready to be collected. The surface is then carefully scraped with a wooden knife. Four crops are generally obtained in a year. The cochineal thus collected is submitted to the action of steam to kill the insect, then dried and packed.

With cochineal, carmin and carmine are prepared:—

Ammonia, in dissolving the coloring matter of the cochineal, completely exhausts the *residuums of cochineal.*

Carmin

Is extracted from cochineal by several processes; we shall describe only that one the most used by perfumers.

Boil one pound of powdered cochineal in ten quarts of water, stir well with a spatula, when the ebullition is too strong pour into the kettle a little cold water. Let it boil for thirty minutes.

Dissolve beforehand one ounce of subcarbonate of soda in one quart of warm water, and pour the solution into the cochineal; stir well and boil a few minutes. Remove from the fire and throw into the kettle one ounce and one drachm of acid sulphate of alumina. Stir well, let it rest from thirty to forty minutes. A red precipitate, composed of alumina and coloring matter, is formed, which is the impure carmin.

Decant into another kettle the red liquid which covers the precipitate. Place this kettle on the fire, pour into it the whites of two eggs well mixed with one pint of water. Stir the liquid briskly. When the ebullition takes place, the white of eggs coagulates and precipitates, carrying with it the coloring matter. Take off from the fire, let it settle half an hour, and decant the liquid. The carmin united to albumen stays at the bottom in the form of a paste. Put this paste in a cloth and let it drain. When it has acquired the consistency of thick cream take it off and spread it on porcelain plates, and dry it in an oven in the dark by a gentle heat.

The residuum left in the first kettle is boiled anew and treated by carbonate of soda. That second operation gives a red liquid which is decanted as the first time, and precipitated by alum. A small quantity of coloring matter is obtained, which can also be employed.

Carmine.

This name has been given to the purified coloring matter of the cochineal. It is very difficult to obtain perfectly pure. The following process is the best:—

Treat powdered cochineal by ether which dissolves the fatty matters it contains; treat afterwards by boiling alcohol, which dissolves the carmine, but deposits it on cooling. The carmine is purified by dissolving it anew in equal parts of alcohol and ether. The carmine deposits slowly in the form of small granules of a fine reddish-purple. Weak acids heighten its odor; alkalies give it a violet shade.

Bresiline,

The coloring matter of *Brazil wood*, is obtained by treating the decoction of this wood by hydrated protoxide of lead and hydrosulphuric acid. If Brazil wood is boiled and perchloride of tin added to the decoction, a fine red precipitate is obtained. If afterwards a certain quantity of acetate of copper is added the red color becomes more intense. The precipitate must be well washed to remove its acid.

Different Forms of Reds (Rouge).

Reds are prepared in different forms—1, powder; 2, pomade; 3, crepons; 4, liquid.

In *powder* it is applied by means of a little plug made of very fine muslin. The *pomade* is applied with the finger and rubbed until well spread, and has no greasy appearance. The *crepons* are pieces of crape saturated with carmine or carthamine, with which the skin is slightly rubbed until the color is uniform. The *liquid* red is the most hurtful to the skin on account of the salts which enter into its composition.

Red with Carmin.

Powdered carmin	. .	2 drachms.
" talc	. . .	4 ounces.

Mix the carmin in a mortar with a little water, introduce the talc, and triturate until a very thick homogeneous paste is obtained; add 10 to 15 drops of a clear solution of gum; then triturating all the time add 6 drops of oil of almonds. Continue to beat until the required consistency is obtained.

Introduce into small porcelain jars and dry in an oven. This red is the brightest; it constitutes the first shade. Other shades may be obtained by changing the proportion of talc.

Second Shade.

For 2 drachms carmine use 4½ ounces talc.

Third Shade.

For 2 drachms carmine use 5 ounces talc, 20 drops of gummy solution, and 8 drops of oil.

Fourth Shade.

For 2 drachms carmine use 5½ ounces talc, 25 drops of gummy solution, and 10 drops of oil. By increasing the proportions of talc, oil, and gummy solution, it is possible to obtain all the shades from the deepest to the lightest.

The red in powder is made in the same manner, only the quantity of oil is diminished, and the gummy solution is dispensed with.

Vegetable Red (in Jars).

Powdered carthamine	.	2 drachms.
" talc .	. .	25 "

Triturate in a mortar with a little distilled water as the above, using the same proportions of gum water and oil.

Liquid Red (No. 1).

Alcohol at 95°	. . .	4 ounces.
Distilled water	. . .	2 "
Carmine	. . . .	¼ drachm.
Aq. ammoniæ	. . .	⅛ "
Oxalic acid	. . .	4½ grains.
Sulphate of alumina	. .	4½ "
Mecca balsam	. . .	4½ "

Dissolve the balsam in a portion of the alcohol, and the carmine in the ammonia, adding a little distilled water; lastly, in a third glass, mix the balance of the alcohol and water, the oxalic acid and sulphate of alumina. When the solution is complete pour in the carmine and balsamic solution; stir, let it settle fifteen minutes, and keep in well-corked bottles.

Another (*No.* 2).

Powdered cochineal	. .	1 ounce.
" cream of tartar	.	1 "
" salts of tartar	.	1 "
" alum	. . .	1 "
Filtered water	. . .	8 ounces.

Boil the cochineal and the salts of tartar in the water; after a few minutes of ebullition add the alum and cream of tartar; pass through a cloth, and put in bottles.

Another (*No.* 3).

Binoxalate of potash	. .	¼ drachm.
Distilled water	. . .	1 pint.
Alcohol	. . . .	1 ounce.
Carmine	. . . .	¼ drachm.
Aqua ammonia	. . .	⅛ "

Dissolve the binoxalate in distilled water, and the carmine in ammonia. Add the alcohol. Mix the whole in a large glass, and stir well.

Different shades may be made with the liquid, and by diluting it with talc, and adding mucilage and a few drops of oil.

First shade:—

Powdered talc	. . .	4 ounces.
Carminated liquor	. .	½ ounce.

Second shade:—

Talc	. . . . .	4 ounces.
Carminated liquor	. .	3 drachms.

Third shade:—

Talc	4 ounces.
Carminated liquor . .	2 drachms.

Fourth shade:—

Talc	4 ounces.
Carminated liquor . .	$1\frac{1}{2}$ drachm.

Dark Red, from Brazil Wood.

Lake of Brazil wood . .	1 pound.
Filtered water . . .	3 pounds.
Lemon juice . . .	q. s.

Dissolve the lake in water; then pour on the lemon juice until the coloring matter is precipitated. Filter, and keep the deposit for future use.

The liquid red is prepared by dissolving this deposit in distilled water.

In jars it is prepared by rubbing this same deposit with talc.

This red is used only on the stage.

SECTION XVII.

SOAPS.

BEFORE the discovery of soap, the cleansing of tissues was effected by argillaceous earths and certain plants, such as the soap-wort, etc. The invention of soap is attributed to the Gauls. They prepared their soap with a lye made from ashes and tallow. The Romans made improvements in its manufacture, and with them it was an important branch of industry. There has been discovered in the ruins of Pompeii a soap manufactory, with all the apparatus, and even tubs full of soap. Others attribute the discovery of soap to the wife of a fisherman in the village of Savona, in the State of Genoa.

Whatever is its origin, this product, as we have seen, was known by the Romans. Modern civilization has perfected its manufacture, and has rendered it absolutely necessary to domestic uses. The word *soap*, chemically speaking, means the body formed by the union of an alkaline, earthy, or metallic oxide, with some of the immediate principles of fatty bodies. In other words, soap is the result of the chemical combination of fatty bodies with alkalies.

Soaps differ from each other according to the nature of the fatty principles which enter into their composition. These principles are *oleine*, *stearine*, *margarine*, *butyrine*, *hyrcine*, *phocenine*, *cetine*, *cholesterine*, and *ethal*.

The different combinations of these principles with alkalies have been divided into four groups.

1. The principles on which the alkalies have no action—*cholesterine* and *ethal*.

2. Those which alkalies transform into *glycerine* and *margaric*, *oleic*, and *stearic acid;* the *stearine*, *oleine*, and *margarine*.

3. Those which alkalies transform into *oleic*, *margaric* acid and *ethal;* *cetine* and *cerine*.

4. Those which on being distilled yield *glycerin*, a *volatile acid*, *oleic* and *margaric* acids; *butyrine*, *phocenine*, and *hyrcine*.

Soaps with soda or potash, furnished by the principles of the second group, are of all these compounds those only which are perfectly soluble in water, and of every-day use. Soda gives hard soap, potash the soft soaps, whatever is the fatty body which enters into their composition.

CHAPTER XXXVII.

PREPARATION OF SOAP.

We have said that every kind of soap is the result of the combination of an alkali with a fatty body; then we must use a fat, and prepare a caustic solution of potash or soda to which has been given the name of *soapmakers' lye.* This lye is prepared as follows:—

Soda or potash	. . .	3 parts.
Water	. . . .	5 "
Quicklime	. . . .	1 "

Dissolve at a gentle heat the alkali in the water; slack the lime separately in an earthen jar, by throwing on it, little by little, water sufficient to reduce it to powder. When the lime is perfectly slacked, pour on it the solution of soda. Stir well and let it settle. Decant the clear liquid, which is the first lye.

The first lye being drawn off, add a new quantity of water, stir well and let it settle, decant the second lye; a third and fourth lye may be obtained in the same manner.

The first lye must mark[1] from 25° to 30°; the

[1] By the hydrometer.

second, from 12° to 18°; the third, from 8° to 10°; the fourth, from 2° to 5°.

These lyes have the property of converting oils and greases into fatty acids, and to form with them oleates, margarates, and stearates of soda or potash perfectly defined. Thus saponification is considered as a true chemical combination, and soap as the intimate union of several salts having the same base.

The lye being prepared, melt slowly in a sheet-iron kettle a certain quantity of pure grease, 100 pounds, for example; when melted pour on it—

Lye at 8° or 10° . . 50 pounds.

Stir all the time with a spatula without boiling. After an hour increase the heat, and when the mass begins to boil refresh it with—

Lye at 15° . . . . 50 pounds.

It is indispensable to pour in the lye by small portions to prevent the mass from boiling over. The saponification is effected, and the soap thus formed is dissolved in water. The solution of soda of a weak degree is used, because at a higher degree the saponification would be imperfect. This first operation is called *saponification.*

To separate the excess of water add little by little a lye of soda containing in solution a strong proportion of kitchen salt. The soap, being insoluble in salt water, soon separates, then the liquid is drawn off, and a new and more concentrated lye containing salt is added. The paste is stirred and kept boiling for some time, then let it settle and draw off the liquid.

Lastly, when the paste is quite homogeneous pour on it—

Lye at 30° . . . 25 pounds.

Heat again and keep boiling for two hours. When the mass does not contain any more free alkali, let it settle and draw off. The operation is then completed. Run the mass into frames which are lined with cotton cloth powdered with a mixture of lime and starch. Next day, remove the soap from the frame and leave it a few days on a table to dry. It is then cut into cakes ready for the perfumer.

CHAPTER XXXVIII.

TOILET SOAPS.

TOILET soaps should be manufactured from materials of the first quality, which, unhappily, is not always the case.

The crude soap being made, it has to be transformed into toilet soap. This transformation requires a series of operations of which we shall give a brief description.

The crude soap is reduced to shavings by means of the cutting machine. These shavings are pressed afterwards between two cylindrical rollers, and are reduced into a thin sheet. This sheet is broken and moistened with rose water, and the soap is passed again through the rollers.

The sheets of soap are divided again with a spatula, and the essences or perfumes are added by small quantities at a time. They are incorporated by stirring well, and the mass is again passed twice through the rollers.

Lastly, take about six pounds of the mass, which is strongly bruised in a marble mortar until it forms a single piece. The mass is then weighed in portions of two, three, and four ounces; they are made into balls on a marble slab, and carried to the drying room. When dried, they are introduced into a copper mould formed of two pieces, and are submitted to the action of a press.

The manner of wrapping soap is not unimportant. If badly wrapped, the perfume evaporates; but if it is put in three envelopes, the first tissue paper, the second tin foil, and the third strong paper, the perfume may be retained a very long time.

Rose Soap.

To one pound of paste of soap incorporate—

Oil of roses . . .	1½ drachm.
" neroli . . .	1 "
" cinnamon . . .	½ "
" geranium . . .	2 drachms.
" bergamot . . .	2 "

Another.

Oil of roses . . .	1 drachm.
" geranium . . .	4 drachms.
" cloves . . .	2 "
" cinnamon . . .	½ drachm.

The soap is colored red with vermilion.

Bitter Almond Soap.

Oil of bitter almonds . .	4 drachms.
" bergamot . . .	6 "

Another.

Oil of mirbane	. . .	6 drachms.
" cinnamon	. . .	$1\frac{1}{4}$ drachm.
" bergamot	. . .	3 drachms.

Orange Flower Soap.

Oil of neroli	. . .	4 drachms.
" geranium	. . .	3 "

Fleurs d'Italie Soap.

Oil of citronella	. . .	3 drachms.
" vervain	. . .	2 "
" mint	. . .	$1\frac{1}{2}$ drachm.

Bouquet des Alpes Soap.

Oil of mint	. . .	2 drachms.
" sage	. . .	2 "
" thyme	. . .	2 "
" lavender	. . .	$1\frac{1}{4}$ drachm.
" rosemary	. . .	$1\frac{1}{4}$ "
" wild thyme	. .	$1\frac{1}{4}$ "

Benzoin Soap.

To twelve pounds of soap paste incorporate—

Tincture of benzoin	. .	1 pound.

Palm Oil Soap.

Oil of cinnamon	. . .	$1\frac{1}{2}$ drachm.
" cloves	. . .	1 "
" lavender	. . .	2 drachms.
" bergamot	. . .	4 "

India Company Soap.

Oil of mace . . .	2 drachms.
" cinnamon . . .	4 "
Balsam of Peru . . .	5 "
Butter of nutmegs . .	1 ounce.

Marshmallow Soap.

Oil of cloves . . .	1¼ drachm.
" cinnamon . . .	½ "
" Portugal . . .	2 drachms.
" thyme . . .	2 "

Vanilla Soap.

To twenty pounds of soap paste incorporate—

Tincture of vanilla . .	1 pound.

Composed Vanilla Soap.

Oil of roses . . .	½ drachm.
Tincture of ambrette . .	1 "
" musk . .	½ "
" vanilla . .	8 ounces.

Patchouly Soap.

Oil of patchouly . .	1¼ drachm.
" bergamot . .	4 drachms.
Tincture of musk . .	½ drachm.

Camphorated Soap.

Oil of almonds . . .	1 ounce.
Tincture of benzoin . .	5 drachms.
Camphor	1¼ drachm.

White Windsor Soap.

Curd soap	10 pounds.
Marine soap . . .	33 ounces.
Oil soap	22 ounces.
Oil of caraway . . .	2½ "
" thyme . . .	2½ "
" rosemary . . .	2½ "
" cassia . . .	4 drachms.
" cloves . . .	4 "

Brown Windsor Soap.

Curd soap	75 pounds.
Marine soap . . .	25 "
Yellow soap . . .	25 "
Oil soap	25 "
Caramel soap . . .	½ pint.
Oil of caraway . . .	2 ounces.
" cloves . . .	2 "
" thyme . . .	2 "
" cassia . . .	2 "
" petit grain . .	2 "
" lavender . . .	2 "

Sand Soap.

Curd soap	7 pounds.
Marine soap . . .	7 "
Sifted white sand . .	28 "
Oil of thyme . . .	2 ounces.
" cassia . . .	2 "
" caraway . . .	2 "
" lavender . . .	2 "

Frangipanni Soap.

Curd soap (previously colored pink)	7 pounds.
Civet	2 drachms.
Oil of neroli	4 "
" sandal	12 "
" rose	2 "
" vitivert	4 "

Citron Soap.

Curd soap	6 pounds.
Oil of citron zest . . .	12 ounces.
" lemon grass . . .	4 drachms.
" bergamot . . .	4 ounces.
" lemon	2 "

Naples Soap.

Butter of cacao	2 drachms.
" nutmegs . . .	2 "
Oil of bergamot . . .	2 "
" cloves	2 "
" neroli	1¼ drachm.
" cherry laurel . . .	1 "
" thyme	1¼ "

Musk Soap.

To 46 pounds of soap paste, and 40 pounds of palm oil soap, incorporate—

Powdered cloves	. .	7 ounces.
" roses	. . .	7 "
" pink	. . .	7 "
Oil of bergamot	. . .	7 "
" musk	. . .	7 "

Honey Soap.

Take five ounces of good Marseilles white soap; five ounces of honey; one ounce of benzoin; four drachms of storax. Mix the whole in a marble mortar; melt over a water bath; pass through a fine silk sieve, and run into a mould.

Light Soap.

It is by beating the soap paste in a kettle that this soap is obtained; salt water is added, and it is again beaten until the paste swells and ascends to the top of the kettle. The more air and water in the paste, the more foamy and light is the soap.

Transparent Soap.

This is manufactured with perfectly dried tallow soap. In the cucurbit of an alembic place equal parts of dry soap and alcohol. Heat over a water bath to 200°. When the solution of the soap is complete, let it settle a few hours; then pour into metallic frames and dry it. This soap acquires all its transparency only after complete desiccation.

To manufacture this soap in small quantity, use the powder of soap treated by an equal weight of alcohol. Dissolve in a small kettle, and after complete solution, run into moulds.

Powder of Soap.

Cut white soap into fine shavings, which are introduced into a dish placed over a water bath heated only to 113° or 122°. Stir all the time till completely dried; reduce it to powder in a mortar, and pass through a fine sieve.

The soap must be perfumed when in paste, for if perfumed while in powder it will not be so white, nor have as agreeable an odor.

Nacreous Soap, or Almond Cream.

If, at the time of the reduction into paste, the soap is strongly ground and beaten for a long time, the paste will take the well-known nacreous appearance. The name of bitter almond cream is due to the fact that it is always perfumed with oil of bitter almonds.

Liquid Soap.

Alcohol	2 quarts.
White powdered soap .	1 pound.
Potash	3½ ounces.

Melt over a water bath, stirring all the time. When dissolved, let it settle, and decant slowly. If the liquid is not clear, it must be filtered; afterwards add oils to perfume it.

Fine Essence of Soap.

Spirit of jasmine . .	8	ounces.
" cassia . . .	8	"
" roses . . .	8	"
" orange flowers .	7	"
" tuberose . .	5	"
" vanilla . .	5	"
" ambrette . .	7	"
Powdered white soap . .	16	"
Potash	5	"
Rose water . . .	8	"

Dissolve the soap and potash in the rose water over a water bath, stirring all the time. When dissolved, stop the heat; mix the spirits well, and pour them into the dish. Carefully mix the soap with the spirits, and when the whole is homogeneous, let it settle, decant, and filter.

SECTION XVIII.

BATHS.

THE use of baths is very ancient, and is found amongst all nations.

It is a natural instinct for man to bathe. The same instinct exists amongst women, who, besides, use the bath as a means of giving brightness and freshness to their skin. It is for this last purpose that *cosmetic* baths have been invented. We shall speak only of the latter, and give the best formulæ.

CHAPTER XXXIX.

COSMETIC BATHS.

THESE baths are generally used for the purpose of keeping or obtaining the polish, brightness, and freshness of the skin. They are prepared by adding to the water of an ordinary bath, substances proper to soften and refresh the cutaneous envelope.

Aromatic and Tonic Bath.

Boil for half an hour in two quarts of fountain water—

Thyme	7 ounces.
Rosemary	10 "
Lavender	8 "
Origanum	7 "
Cloves	10 cloves.
Nutmegs	5 nutmegs.

Remove from the fire, and throw the decoction into an ordinary bath.

Another.

Thyme	7 ounces.
Lavender	7 "
Marjoram	5 "
Sage	5 "
Fennel	5 "
Mint	7 "
Parsley	5 "
Origanum	7 "
Wormwood . . .	5 "

Boil in a kettle with—

Fountain water . . .	6 quarts.
Red wine	5 "

After an ebullition of half an hour, pass through a fine sieve and throw the decoction into an ordinary bath.

Aromatic Sachet for Bath.

Fill a bag of thin cotton cloth with powdered nutmegs and cloves, orange peel, dried rose and violet leaves, mint, lavender, laurel, orris-root, and anis.

Place the bag in the bath-tub under warm water. When the tub is one-third full, stir the water and press the bag. After a quarter of an hour reduce the bath to the required temperature with cold water.

Raspail's Alkaline Bath.

Ammonia saturated with camphor	7 ounces.
Kitchen salt	2 pounds.

First pour into the bath-tub two or three pails of water, then pour in the solution of ammonia and salt, fill the tub with water, stir well.

Artificial Sea-Water Bath.

Kitchen salt . . .	4 pounds.
Sulphate of soda . .	2 "
Chloride of magnesium .	2 "
" calcium . .	1 pound.

Dissolve in a bath of 25 gallons of water.

Sulphurous Bath.

Sulphuret of potassium .	4 ounces.
Water	1 pound.

Dissolve and filter, then add to the water of the bath.

Alkaline Bath to Cleanse the Skin.

Ordinary carbonate of soda 10 ounces.

Dissolve in a quart of warm water and pour into a bath of 32 gallons of water.

Soapy Bath.

Soap . . . . . . 2 pounds.
Soda . . . . . . 7 ounces.

Reduce the soap to shavings and introduce it into a kettle with 3 quarts of water; heat gently. To facilitate the solution add from time to time the soda previously dissolved in water. Stir until all the soap is dissolved. Add the remainder of the soda and pour the whole into an ordinary bath.

Emollient Bath to Soften the Skin.

Pearl barley . . . . 1 pound.
Hulled rice . . . . 8 ounces.
Bran . . . . . . 4 pounds.
Borage . . . . . 4 handfuls.
Flowers of malva . . . 4 "
" white sage . . 4 "
Linseed . . . . . 8 ounces.

Boil in a sufficient quantity of water. With the decoction prepare a bath.

Another.

Emollient plants . . . 4 pounds.
Linseed . . . . . 8 ounces.

Boil in one gallon of water, pass through a sieve, then pour into the bath. Stir well.

Bath of Beauty, called Ninon de Lenclos' Bath.

In 1 quart of water dissolve—

Kitchen salt . . .	8 ounces.
Carbonate of soda . .	3½ "

In 3 quarts of milk dissolve—

Honey	3 pounds.

Pour the first solution into the bath and stir well. Then pour in the mixture of honey and milk, stir well, and the bath is ready.

Another, used in Persia.

Pearl barley . . .	3 pounds.
Powdered lupuline . .	2 "
Rice	1 pound.
Borage	1 "
Rosemary and angelica, each	1 "

Boil in a sufficient quantity of water and throw into an ordinary bath.

Aromatic Gelatinous Bath.

Aromatized gelatine . .	1 pound.
Kitchen salt . . .	5 ounces.
Dissolved white soap . .	1 pound.

Dissolve in—

Boiling water . . .	2 gallons.

Mix with the bath.

Modesty Bath.

Sweet almonds	. . .	8 ounces.
Enula campana	. . .	4 "
Linseed flour	. . .	8 "
Buckwheat flour	. .	1 pound.

Rub these substances together in a mortar and reduce them to a paste, by adding water rendered milky by the addition of a little tincture of benzoin, then form three bags, one large and two small. Use them while in the bath.

Scented Bath.

Strawberries	. . .	15 pounds.
Raspberries	. . .	5 "
Bran	. . . . .	5 "
Malva powder	. . .	2 "

Rub in a mortar, moistening with—

Rose water	. . . .	8 ounces.

When the whole is reduced to a paste, throw it into the empty tub, then dilute it by pouring on it by degrees the water of the bath. When perfectly diluted, pour all the necessary water, stir well, and the bath is ready.

Perfumed Baths.

These kinds of bath are prepared by adding to the water of an ordinary bath perfumes according to the taste. The following formula is an example:—

Rose water	3 pints.
Tincture of benzoin . .	2 ounces.
Essence of thyme . .	1 ounce.
Cologne water . . .	2 ounces.

Stir the mixture with the water of the bath for a few minutes.

Milk Baths.

The use of these baths is rare on account of their cost. They could be substituted by mixing with the water of an ordinary bath a decoction of 8 pounds of malva leaves, 8 ounces of hyssop, and 2 pounds of bran. This bath acquires more prominence, softening and cosmetic properties, if to the decoction one pound of gelatine is added.

SECTION XIX.

HAIR DYES.

The hair is formed of two parts: an outside, tubulous envelope, which is colorless; and inside, a horny substance more or less colored reddish, black, flaxen, or chestnut, which gives the shade to the hair. Grief, excesses, etc., dry the root of the hairs, and are the cause of their falling. Hairs may be kept without alteration for centuries. The analysis of black hair, as given by Vauquelin, is as follows:—

An animal substance,
A white concrete oil,
A greenish-black oil,
Oxide of iron,
Oxide of manganese,
Phosphate of lime,
Carbonate of lime,
Silica,
Sulphur.

Red hair has the same composition, except that the *oily substance* is red.

White hair, beside the above constituents, contains *phosphate of magnesia.* There is no positive age at which the hair begins to grow white, but it has been remarked that it is between 35 and 40 years of age that this phenomenon begins to appear. The color of the hair has a great influence on the period when decoloration begins. Black hair whitens quicker than the flaxen.

Diseases, deep griefs, mental troubles, excess in pleasures, etc., often advance the time of the decoloration of the hair. Certain skin diseases also determine a change in the color; this phenomenon is caused by the alteration of the hair bulbs. Whatever is the state of decoloration, its cause always resides in the bulb, and is determined by the suppression of the secretion of the colored animal oil which gives to the hair its different shades.

The color of the hair may be artifically changed. The dyeing in black is a common thing, but a fact which is not generally known is that with chlorinated water black hair can be transformed into red and flaxen.

Generally all the preparations used to dye the hair are more or less dangerous, because they contain corrosive substances which dry or burn the root, and also irritate the skin, and by their absorption produce bad effects on the health. They are always salts of silver, lead, bismuth, or mercury; with nitric, sulphuric, or sulphidic acids; lime, potash, etc. etc., substances the very names of which would indicate the danger of their use. Medical works are full of cases of accidents produced by these preparations, and we call the attention of the reader to the fact that sooner or later their effects will be revealed in the system.

CHAPTER XL.

FORMULÆ FOR HAIR-DYES.

Ordinary Process.

Powdered minium . .	1 ounce.
Hydrated lime . . .	4 ounces.

Mix well; moisten the mixture with a weak solution of potash, so as to make a thin paste.

China Water.

Nitrate of silver . . .	1 ounce.
Hydrated lime . . .	4 ounces.

Dissolve in a sufficient quantity of water, and filter. This solution gives a black with reddish reflection; it alters the hair, which becomes red after some time.

Berzelius' Process.

Nitrate of silver . . .	1 ounce.
Slaked lime . . .	2 ounces.

Grind the nitrate and the lime; add a little oil or pomade; grind again until perfectly mixed. The fatty body is added to prevent the blackening action of the nitrate on the skin.

Paste to Blacken the Hair.

Nitrate of silver . . .	½	ounce.
Protonitrate of mercury .	½	"
Distilled water	4½	ounces.

Dissolve and filter. Wash the deposit with enough water to obtain 5½ ounces of solution. Prepare with this solution and a little starch a half-fluid paste, with which the hair is to be rubbed. Cover the head immediately with a cap of water-proof cloth. The application is made at night; next morning wash the hair, dry, and oil.

Hahnemann's Powder.

Powdered litharge . .	8	ounces.
Slaked lime	4	"
Powdered starch . .	2	"

Apply as the above. This process is very dangerous.

Another.

Acetate of lead	2	ounces.
Carbonate of lime . .	3	"
Slaked lime	4	"
Soda	2	"

Apply as the above. Dangerous to use.

Egyptian Water.

Nitrate of silver	1	ounce.
" bismuth . .	1	"
Subacetate of lead . .	4	ounces.

Dissolve in a sufficient quantity of warm water, and with a sponge dampen the hair. One hour after, dip another sponge in concentrated sulphuretted water, and pass it over the hair, which becomes black immediately. Very dangerous.

Tincture with Plumbite of Lime.

Sulphate of lead . .	4	ounces.
Hydrated lime . . .	4	"
Water	30	"

Boil an hour and a quarter, and filter. During the ebullition the lime combines with sulphuric acid, and the oxide of lead set free unites with the excess of lime.

This preparation gives a black with a red reflection.

Jouvence Water

Is compounded in two bottles.

First Bottle.—

Nitrate of silver . . .	4	ounces.
Distilled water . . .	20	"

Some color the solution blue with a little nitrate of copper, and some color it yellow with chromate of potash; while others color green, rose, etc.

Second Bottle.—The object of the liquor of this bottle is to sulphurize or blacken the silver solution.

Sulphydric acid or sulphide of potassium dissolved in water, or—

Sulphydrate of ammonia	.	1 ounce.
Solution of potash	. .	3 drachms.
Distilled water	. . .	1 ounce.

The hair is first moistened with solution No. 1; one hour after, it is treated with solution No. 2, and immediately a sulphide of silver is formed round the hair. Sometimes the black is greenish, sometimes reddish. This preparation quickly destroys the hair.

English Tincture.

Green shells of walnuts	.	5 ounces.
Litharge	. . . .	2 "
Slaked lime	. . .	2 "

The color obtained is that of soot.

Argentic Pomade.

Nitrate of silver	. . .	2 drachms.
Cream tartar	. . .	2 "
Ammonia	. . . .	4 "
Lard	. . . . .	4 "

Prepare in a glass mortar. This pomade is applied with a brush. It gives a very poor black.

Argentic Tincture.

First Bottle.—Concentrated solution of bichloride of tin.

Second Bottle.—Diluted solution of nitrate of silver.

It gives a fine black, but becomes reddish in a short time.

Vegetable Tincture.

Green shells of walnuts .	4 ounces.
Red wine	7 "

American Process.

Nitrate of silver . . .	1 ounce.
" bismuth . .	1 "
Distilled water . . .	6 ounces.

Moisten the hair with this solution. One hour after, touch with sulphydric acid.

Pomade to Dye the Hair.

Beef marrow . . .	3½ ounces.
White wax . . .	1 ounce.
Nitrate of silver . . .	½ drachm.

Melt these substances together over a water bath, and add to them plumbago in sufficient quantity to obtain the required shade.

Soap to Render the Hair Black.

Tallow	2 ounces.
Liquid pitch . . .	1 ounce.
Powdered plumbago . .	½ "
Labdanum	½ "
Varnish	½ "

Mix, and add—

Lye of ashes . . a sufficient quantity.

Flaxen Dye.

Acetate of iron	1 ounce.
Nitrate of bismuth	2 ounces.
" silver	1 ounce.
Distilled water	10 ounces.

Another.

Protochloride of tin	2 ounces.
Hydrated lime	3 "

Moisten the hair with either of these two preparations; one hour after, touch it with a mixture of equal parts of distilled water and sulphide of potassium.

Cosmetic to Prevent Baldness.

Medicated soap	1 ounce.
Leather ashes	1 "
Salt	1 "
Red tartar	1 "
Hair powder	1 "
Sulphate of iron	2 drachms.
Sal ammoniac	2 "
Colocynth	2 "
Catechu	2 "

Mix; add lard enough to make a pomade.

Conservative Water for the Hair.

Rum	1 pint.
White wine	4 pints.
Decoction of barley	1 pint.

Fluid of Java for Reviving the Bulbs.

Beef marrow	2 ounces.
White wax	1½ ounce.
Olive oil	2 ounces.

Tincture for Baldness.

Cherry-laurel leaves . .	2 ounces.
Cloves	2 drachms.
Alcoholate of lavender .	6 ounces.
" origanum .	6 "

Digest for six days, press, and to the filtrate add—

Sulphuric ether . . . ½ ounce.

Keep in ground-stoppered bottles.

Bandolines.

The liquid bandolines are principally of a gummy nature, being made either with Iceland moss or linseed and water, variously perfumed, or by boiling quince-seed with water. Perfumers, however, chiefly make bandoline from gum tragacanth.

Rose Bandoline.

Gum tragacanth . . .	6 ounces.
Rose water . . .	1 gallon.
Oil of roses . . .	4 drachms.

Steep the gum in the water for twenty-four or thirty-six hours; as it swells and forms a gelatinous mass, it should be stirred from time to time. It is then squeezed through a linen cloth and allowed to stand for a few days, and passed through a cloth a second time; when the oil is thoroughly incorporated.

Almond Bandoline

Is made as the above, scenting with two drachms of oil of almonds in place of the roses.

Crême de Mauve, or Hair-Gloss.

Pure glycerine . . .	4 pounds.
Spirit of jasmine . .	1 pint.
Aniline	5 drops.

CHAPTER XLI.

ECONOMICAL SCENTS—FLAVORING EXTRACTS.

Economical Scents.

As cheap perfumes are often required to fill little fancy bottles, the following recipes for their manufacture will be found of service:—

I.	Spirit of wine . . .	1 pint.
	Essence of bergamot .	1 ounce.
II.	Spirit of wine . . .	1 pint.
	Oil of sandal . . .	1 ounce.
III.	Spirit of wine . . .	1 pint.
	Oil of lavender . . .	4 drachms.
	" bergamot . .	4 "
	" cloves . . .	1 drachm.
IV.	Spirit of wine . . .	1 pint.
	Oil of lemon grass . .	2 drachms.
	Essence of lemons . .	4 "
V.	Spirit of wine . . .	1 pint.
	Oil of petit grain . .	2 drachms.
	" orange peel . .	4 "

These mixtures are to be filtered through paper, with the addition of a little magnesia to make them bright.

Flavoring Extracts.

Prof. W. Procter, Jr., of Philadelphia, has published in the *American Journal of Pharmacy* several formulæ for the manufacture of these extracts; and as we consider them the best, we think it will interest the reader to know their preparation.

Lemon.

Exterior rinds of lemons .	4 ounces.
Deodorized alcohol at 95° .	2 quarts.
Recent oil of lemon . .	6 ounces.

Expose the rind to the air until partially dry; bruise it in a wedgewood mortar; add it to the alcohol, with agitation until the color is extracted. Add the oil; and if it does not immediately dissolve and become clear, let it stand for a day or two, agitating occasionally. Filter.

Orange.

Exterior rind of fresh oranges	4 ounces.
Deodorized alcohol at 95° .	1 quart.
Recent oil of orange . .	2 ounces.

Operate as for the lemon.

Bitter Almonds.

Oil of bitter almonds . .	4 ounces.
Alcohol at 95° . . .	1 quart.
Tincture of turmeric . .	1 ounce.

Mix.

As this extract in quantity is poisonous, it is better to deprive it of its hydrocyanic acid as follows:—

Oil of bitter almonds . .	4 ounces.
Sulphate of iron . .	2 "
Lime recently burned .	1 ounce.
Water . . .	a sufficient quantity.

Dissolve the iron in a pint of water, and slake the lime with another pint; mix them together, and shake that mixture with the oil. Distil in a glass retort until the whole of the oil has passed over. The oil, after allowing time to separate from the water, is removed for use.

Rose.

Oil of rose . . .	1 drachm.
Hundred-leaved roses . .	2 ounces.
Deodorized alcohol . .	1 quart.

Bruise the leaves. Make an extract from them by maceration in alcohol; press so as to get one quart, in which the oil is dissolved; filter through paper. If there are no rose leaves, add a minute quantity of tincture of cochineal, to give a pale rose tint.

Cinnamon.

Oil of cinnamon . .	2 drachms.
Powdered Ceylon cinnamon	4 ounces.
Deodorized alcohol . .	1 pint.
Water	1 "

Dissolve the oil in the alcohol, and gradually add the water and then the cinnamon; agitate several hours; filter through paper.

Nutmegs.

Oil of nutmegs . . .	2 drachms.
Powdered mace . . .	1 ounce.
Deodorized alcohol . .	1 quart.

Mix the oil and mace together, add the alcohol, macerate twelve hours, and filter.

Ginger.

Powdered ginger . .	4 ounces.
Deodorized alcohol .	a sufficient quantity.
Syrup	8 ounces.

Pack the ginger in a percolator, moisten it with a little alcohol, then pour on alcohol until 1½ pint of tincture has passed. Add the syrup, and mix.

Black Pepper and Capsicum.—These are made from powdered pepper and capsicum in the same manner as ginger, except that the syrup is omitted, and enough alcohol is used to make one quart.

Coriander.

Powdered coriander . .	4 ounces.
Oil of coriander . . .	1 drachm.
Alcohol at 95° . . .	1½ pint.
Water	½ "

Mix the alcohol and water, add the coriander previously mixed with the oil. Macerate twenty-four hours, decant the liquid, put in a percolator, pour on the decanted liquid, add alcohol enough to make one quart.

Vanilla.

Vanilla	1 ounce.
Sugar	2 ounces.
Syrup	1 pint.
Diluted alcohol	a sufficient quantity.

Cut the vanilla into small pieces and triturate it with sugar until in coarse powder, put in a percolator, pour in the alcohol until one pint has been drawn off, add the syrup, and mix.

Celery.

Celery seeds	2 ounces.
Deodorized alcohol	a sufficient quantity.
Water	a sufficient quantity.

Bruise the seeds, percolate with alcohol one pint, add water until one pint has been drawn off; mix; triturate with one drachm of carbonate of magnesia; filter.

Soup Herbs.

Thyme	1 ounce.
Sweet marjoram	1 "
" basil	1 "
Summer savory	1 "
Celery seeds	1 drachm.

Percolate with diluted alcohol sufficient to make one pint.

CHAPTER XLII.

NEW AND PERFECTED PRODUCTS.

Crême-neige (*Snow-Cream*).

Spermaceti	3	ounces.
White wax	2	"
Fresh oil of almonds	12	"

Melt over a water bath and pour into a marble mortar. Stir the mass quickly with an ivory spatula, so as to prevent the formation of grains. When the mass has a buttery consistency triturate with the pestle, beat well for fifteen or twenty minutes, being careful to scrape with the spatula all the parts which have not been ground by the pestle. When a kind of white cream has been obtained, add, little by little, stirring all the time—

Double water of roses	1	ounce.
White and odorless glycerine	1	"

Beat twenty minutes to incorporate, and add—

Pure essence of roses	10	drops.

Beat again quickly for thirty or forty minutes, then a white cream with a very sweet odor is obtained. Fill porcelain jars with it, and paste a thin band of paper round the edge of the cover. The more this cream is beaten the longer it keeps.

This preparation is one of the most pleasant cosmetics for the skin.

Pommade Trikophile.

Pure and odorless veal grease	6½ ounces.
Spermaceti	3¼ "
White wax	1 ounce.
Oil of bitter almonds . .	8 ounces.

Melt together over a water bath and pour into a marble mortar, beat as indicated in the above preparation until a smooth paste, without grains, is obtained. Perfume the pomade by adding essences according to taste.

This pomade may be employed as an excipient for different tonic and fortifying substances, such as balsams, extract of cinchona, tannin, etc., prescribed in atony of the skin of the head.

Brillantine.

Pure veal grease . .	3½ ounces.
Spermaceti	3½ "
White wax	1 ounce.
Oil of almonds . . .	3½ ounces.

Melt over a water bath and beat as above. Afterwards pour in—

Castor oil	2 ounces.

Beat to incorporate, then add concentrated solution of gum tragacanth in two ounces of rose water. Beat anew until perfectly incorporated, then aromatize according to taste.

Pommade Souveraine to Prevent the Fall of the Hair.

Pure veal grease . .	8 ounces.
Nerval balsam . . .	$3\frac{1}{2}$ "
Oil of almonds . . .	5 "

Melt over a water bath, pour into a marble mortar, and beat well so as to obtain a homogeneous paste. In a porcelain dish melt—

Subcarbonate of soda . .	16 ounces.
Kitchen salt . . .	2 "
Alcohol	1 ounce.
Distilled water . . .	2 ounces.

Pour this solution over the pomade and triturate until well incorporated. Aromatize according to taste.

Another.

Pure veal grease . .	16 ounces.
Soft soap	2 "
Kitchen salt . . .	1 ounce.
Nerval balsam . . .	2 ounces.

Over a water bath melt the balsam, grease, and soap, pour into a mortar and beat, adding at the same time a little oil of almonds. Dissolve the kitchen salt in tepid rose water; when dissolved pour into the mortar. Triturate till perfectly incorporated.

Sulphuretted Pomade (for itching of the head).

Pure veal grease . .	13½ ounces.
Crême-neige . . .	3½ "
Washed sulphur . .	3½ "
Subcarbonate of soda .	2½ "
Oil of bitter almonds .	3½ "

Triturate in a mortar the sulphur and crême-neige; dissolve the soda in 2 ounces of laurel water; and pour the solution on the sulphur; triturate thoroughly. Place the grease and oil over a water bath, and when melted pour them into the mortar with the other ingredients; beat until a homogeneous pomade is obtained. Perfume according to taste. Rub the head with this pomade, and in a few days the itching will disappear.

Pomade Trikogene (for incipient baldness).

Pure veal grease . .	12 ounces.
Nerval balsam . . .	5 "
Nutmeg butter . . .	5 "
Oil of almonds . . .	6½ "

Melt and beat as above, then add—

Croton oil	10 drops.

Beat to incorporate.

In another vessel dissolve:—

Subcarbonate of soda . .	3½ ounces.
Distilled water . . .	1 ounce.
Alcohol	1 "

Pour the solution over the pomade and triturate until perfectly incorporated. Aromatize according to taste.

Ferruginous Pomade (*tonic and astringent*).

Pure veal grease . . .	8 ounces.
Spermaceti	8 "
White wax . . .	2 "
Oil of almonds . . .	10 "

Melt and beat as above.

In a porcelain dish dissolve:—

Distilled water . . .	1⅛ ounce.
Sulphate of iron . .	6 drachms.

Pour the solution over the pomade and beat to incorporate.

Add afterwards the following solution:—

Gallic acid	6 drachms.
Water and alcohol, of each	6 "

Pour the solution into the mortar by small quantities at a time and triturate until you have a homogeneous paste of a grayish-blue color. Perfume to taste.

By increasing the dose of iron and gallic acid a black pomade is obtained; on the contrary, by diminishing them, the color takes a lighter shade.

Detersive Lotion (*for fall of the hair*).

Alcoholate of soap . .	16 ounces.
Subcarbonate of soda . .	3½ "
Camphorated alcohol . .	4 "

Dissolve the soda, and filter until the liquor is clear.

Another.

Red wine	16 ounces.
Kitchen salt . . .	1 ounce.
Tannin	2½ drachms.

Dissolve and filter.

Alcoholate of Soap (to cleanse the head).

Marseilles soap . . .	10 ounces.
Filtered water . . .	23½ "
Subcarbonate of soda .	3½ "

Dissolve with a gentle heat, stirring all the time. When the solution is complete, stop the heat, let it cool a little, and add—

Alcohol at 80° . . .	1 pint.

Stir to incorporate; aromatize, and filter until perfectly clear.

Sulphurous Iodized Lotion (for scurf and freckles).

Concentrated solution of sulphide of potassium	8 ounces.
Solution of hydrosulphate of ammonia	2 "

Mix in a large glass. Then add—

Ioduretted iodide solution .	3½ ounces.

Let it settle. A deposit is formed, decant and filter. Pour in ground-stoppered bottles and keep for use.

Callidermic Lotion (to render the skin healthy).

First Vial.

Hyposulphite of soda .	8 ounces.
Ioduretted iodide solution .	3½ "

Dissolve the hyposulphite in 23½ ounces of filtered water, then add the iodide. If the liquor is reddish, add a little hyposulphite, to decolorize.

Second Vial.

Sulphide of potassium .	2 ounces.
Filtered water . . .	8 "
Essence of lemon . .	5 drops.

Mix and stir.

These two liquids must be filtered several times.

Application.—Fill a glass three-fourths full with preparation No. 1; pour in afterwards, drop by drop, the liquor No. 2, until a yellowish milk is obtained. Wash the face with a cloth which has been dipped in the preparation.

Ioduretted Iodide Solution.

Tincture of iodine . .	4 drachms.
Iodide of potassium . .	5 "
Filtered water . . .	3½ ounces.

Mix.

Cosmetic Lotion.

Rose water . . .	8 ounces.
Cherry-laurel water . .	8 "
Cacao butter . . .	3½ "
Cream of soap . . .	5 drachms.
Benzoic acid . . .	1 drachm.

Triturate in a marble mortar the butter and soap. Add, little by little, the rose water. Dissolve the benzoic acid in a little alcohol, and pour into the mortar. Add afterwards the laurel water; beat well, to mix all the ingredients.

Callidermic Powder (*to refresh and whiten the skin*).

Finely-powdered marshmallow	8 ounces.
Rye flour	3½ "
Dextrine	2 "

Mix, and pass through a sieve.

At night, before going to bed, make a paste by mixing the powder with a sufficient quantity of water of bitter almonds. Cover the face with the paste so as to form a thin coating. Next day remove it with tepid water, and wash well.

Callidermic Paste.

Cream of soap . . .	8 ounces.
Honey	13½ "
Oil of bitter almonds . .	13½ "
Almond flour . . .	5 "
Glycerine	3½ "
Rose water	3½ "
White silica in jelly . .	3½ "

This paste should be white, homogeneous, free from grains, and half fluid. It is perfumed according to taste.

Preparation of Silica.

White sand . . .	1 pound.
Anhydrous soda . . .	3 pounds.

Mix these two substances together, introduce them into a crucible, heat in a reverberatory furnace until the mass is melted and vitrified. Break the crucible so as to collect the product, which is a silicate of soda. Reduce it to a coarse powder, which is introduced into a porcelain dish filled with water; boil so as to make a solution of the silicate, also called *fusible glass.* When the whole is dissolved, decant into an earthen jar, and let it cool. Take water acidulated with sulphuric or hydrochloric acid, pour slowly this acidulated water into the solution of silicate of soda, and stir the whole with a glass rod. Very soon the liquid is transformed into a jelly, which is collected on a cloth filter, and suffered to drain. Put the jelly into a clean earthen jar, and wash it with water until it is no longer acid; filter it, and let it drain. After ten or twelve hours, press the filter, and keep the jelly in porcelain jars.

Hydrated silica is used to prepare the callidermic paste and the dermophile soap. Dried and reduced into a very fine powder, it enters into the composition of *callidermic whites.*

Preparation of Talc.

Take powdered talc, pass it through a fine sieve, then throw the sifted powder into a dishful of water, and stir well with a spatula. Pass the water through a coarse cloth, and let it settle. The talc in suspension falls to the bottom in an impalpable powder. Decant the clear water, and pour the paste on pieces of paper; place them in an oven, and let them dry. After desiccation, introduce into a mortar, powder, and pass through a fine silk sieve. A superior powder of talc is thus obtained.

New White in Powder.

Silica in fine powder . .	3½ ounces.
Talc in fine powder . .	2 "
Washed oxide of zinc .	1 ounce.
Powdered starch . .	1 "

Mix, pass through a fine silk sieve, and keep in boxes.

New White (Liquid).

Silica in fine powder . .	2 ounces.
Oxide of zinc ground with water	10 "
Powdered talc . . .	1 ounce.
Filtered water . . .	23½ ounces.

Mix in a mortar and keep in bottles for use.

New White (Plastic).

Oxide of zinc . . .	16 ounces.
Powdered talc . . .	2½ "
Soap-water	32 ounces.

Mix in a mortar and pour into bottles.

White in Trochists.

Oxide of zinc ground in water	16 ounces.
Filtered talc . . .	5 "

Soap-water, slightly gummy, a sufficient quantity. Rub in a mortar, watering little by little with the soapy water until a homogeneous paste is obtained, then mould the white in sticks.

Dermophile Soap.

To the paste of ordinary soap add fifteen per cent. of hydrated silica, and stir the paste well so as to incorporate the silica; mould and dry.

Cyanuretted Pomade.

Snow cream (crême-neige) .	3½ ounces.
Oxide of zinc . . .	1 ounce.
Cyanide of potassium .	7 grains.

Triturate the oxide of zinc with the cream; dissolve the cyanide in distilled rose water, and pour into the pomade; beat until well incorporated.

Milk of Roses.

Almonds	8 ounces.
Rose water	2 quarts.
Cream of soap . . .	2 ounces.
Spermaceti	1 ounce.
Almond oil . . .	2 ounces.
Alcohol	13½ "

Essence of bergamot . .	½ ounce.
" rose . . .	1 drachm.
Tincture of musked amber .	1 "
" benzoin . .	4 drachms.

Prepare an emulsion by grinding the almonds with the rose water; pass through a sieve. Melt the spermaceti and the cream in the oil and introduce into a marble mortar; beat, adding little by little the emulsion, until a perfectly homogeneous liquid without grains is obtained. Add the essences and tinctures; triturate anew until perfectly incorporated.

Philodontine Water.

Cloves	1 ounce.
Cinnamon	1 "
Anise	1 "
Guaiacum	1 "
Cinchona	1 "
Powdered catechu . .	1 "
Cubebs	½ "

Macerate for fifteen days in one quart of alcohol at 59°. Filter, and add—

Alcoholate of pyrethrum .	7 ounces.
Peppermint water . .	7 "
Oil of peppermint . .	1 ounce.

The oil of peppermint has previously been dissolved in five ounces of alcohol. If a pink color is required, triturate half an ounce cochineal with one ounce cream tartar in a sufficient quantity of warm water, pour into the mass, stir well, and filter a second time.

This preparation is used to wash the teeth and mouth.

Hesperides Water.

Essence of	bergamot	½ ounce.
"	lemon	½ "
"	Portugal	½ "
"	cedrat	5 drachms.
"	cloves	1 drachm.
"	carvi	½ "
"	white thyme	2½ drachms.
"	vervain	4 "
"	lavender	5 "
"	white geranium	1 drachm.
"	roses	¼ "
"	anise	1 "
Tincture of	ambrette	3½ ounces.
"	Tolu	2 "
"	musk	2½ drachms.
Essence of	peppermint	2½ "
Alcohol at 95°		2 quarts.

Pour the whole into a bottle of three quarts capacity, stir quickly to mix well, let it stand several hours, and filter until clear.

If, instead of filtering, you distil so as to extract three pints of product, a much finer and sweeter aromatic water is obtained.

Lactated Bath (*Artificial Milk Bath*).

Into a marble mortar introduce—

Cream of soap . . .	8 ounces.
White honey . . .	5 "
Solution of carbonate of soda	3½ "

Triturate until a thin paste is obtained, then add—

Sifted almond flour . .	2½ ounces.
Oil of almonds . . .	2 "

Triturate to incorporate, and aromatize with—

Tincture of Tolu . .	6 drachms.
" benzoin . .	6 "
Essence of lavender . .	4 "
" thyme . .	2½ "
" vervain . .	2½ "

Beat until completely incorporated, and if the paste is too thick, add distilled rose water to render it half-fluid. Pour into wide mouthed bottles of one pint capacity, and keep for use.

Before using, dip the bottle in warm water, to liquefy the product, and mix in the water of the bath.

Water for Bad Breath.

Chloride of lime . . .	½ drachm.
Fountain water . . .	1 quart.

Dissolve, filter, and add—

Essence of peppermint .	1 ounce.
Sugar	7 ounces.

Wash the mouth with this water, which corrects the offensive breath.

Disinfecting Lozenges.

Catechu	1 ounce.
Magnesia	½ "
Sugar	4 ounces.
Essence of lemon . .	20 drops.
" cinnamon . .	20 "
" peppermint .	20 "
Mucilage	s. q.

Make lozenges weighing fifteen grains. They are used to remove the fetidity of the stomach.

Balsamic Tincture (for the teeth).

Catechu	1 ounce.
Myrrh	1 "
Balsam of Peru . . .	1 drachm.
Alcoholate of cochlearia .	4 ounces.

Reduce these substances to a fine powder, and macerate them for six days in the alcohol. Filter.

This tincture is the best to use to give a healthy tone to the gums. One spoonful of it in half a tumbler of water is sufficient to rinse the mouth.

Pommade Rosat (for chapped lips, hands, etc.).

Oil of sweet almonds . .	2 ounces.
White wax . . .	1½ drachm.
Spermaceti . . .	2½ drachms.
Alkanet root . . .	2½ "

Heat over a water bath until melted, pour into a mortar, stirring with a wooden pestle, and add—

Rose water . . .	2½ drachms.
Sulphate of zinc . .	1¼ drachm.

The sulphate of zinc is previously dissolved in a little rose water. Beat the mixture until the whole is incorporated, aromatize with a few drops of rose oil, and then put in jars for use.

Pomade for Piles.

Populeum ointment . .	2 ounces.
Althea " . . .	2 "
Pommade rosat . . .	2 "
White honey . . .	1 ounce.
Oil of sweet almonds . .	1 "

Melt over a water bath, and triturate in a marble mortar, with the addition of a few drops of laudanum.

Pomade for Chapped Hands.

Chloride of lime . . .	1 drachm.
New lard	1 ounce.

After trituration, incorporate—

Tannin	¼ drachm.

Rub morning and night.

Another.

Fresh cold cream . .	1 ounce.
Gallic acid	½ drachm.
Water of bitter almonds .	4 drachms.

Triturate until the mass is homogeneous.

Balsam for Chapped Hands.

Tincture of benzoin . .	½ ounce.
Camphor	¾ drachm.

Dissolve by triturating in a porcelain mortar; then add—

Crême-neige . . .	1 ounce.
Tannin	½ drachm.

Triturate until well incorporated, and aromatize with oil of bergamot.

English Vinegar.

Pure acetic acid . . .	16 ounces.
Camphor	2 "
Oil of cloves . . .	2 drachms.
" cinnamon . .	1¼ drachm.
" bergamot . . .	2½ drachms.
Tincture of ambergris and musk	¼ drachm.

Mix and filter. Pour into small vials filled beforehand with crystals of sulphate of potash.

Ethereal Aromatic Tincture.

Cinnamon	1¼ drachm.
Cloves	2½ drachms.
Nutmegs	2½ "
Vanilla	1¼ drachm.
Musk	¼ drachm.
Alcohol at 95° . . .	16 ounces.

Macerate eight days, then add—

Ether	5 ounces.

Leave for a few hours, filter, and keep in ground-stoppered vials.

Water for Headache.

Aqua ammonia . . .	1 ounce.
Oil of wild thyme . .	½ "
" carvi . . .	½ "
Camphorated brandy . .	5 ounces.
English vinegar . . .	3½ "

Mix and allow to stand a few hours, and filter; to the filtrate add—

Acetic ether . . .	2½ drachms.

Stir, and keep in ground-stoppered bottles.

Vulnerary Water.

Melissa	1 handful.
Mint	1 "
Sage	1 "
Wild thyme . . .	1 "
Wormwood . . .	1 "
Marjoram	1 "
Sweet basil . . .	1 "

Macerate the plants in—

Alcohol	2 quarts.

Express and add—

Soapy alcohol . . .	8 ounces.
Tincture of lavender . .	8 "

Filter.

Ethereal Aromatic Tincture.

Cloves	2½ drachms.
Cinnamon	2½ "
Ginger	1¼ drachm.
Cardamom seeds . . .	1¼ "
Balsam of Tolu . . .	2½ drachms.
Castor	½ drachm.
Ether	16 ounces.

Macerate a few days in a corked bottle, then add—

Alcoholate of melissa	8 ounces.

Shake and filter.

INDEX.

THE END.

CATALOGUE

OF

PRACTICAL AND SCIENTIFIC BOOKS,

PUBLISHED BY

HENRY CAREY BAIRD,

INDUSTRIAL PUBLISHER,

No. 406 WALNUT STREET,

PHILADELPHIA.

☞ Any of the Books comprised in this Catalogue will be sent by mail, free of postage, at the publication price.

☞ My New and Enlarged Catalogue, 82 pages 8vo., with full descriptions of Books, will be sent, free of postage, to any one who will favor me with his address.

ARMENGAUD, AMOUROUX, AND JOHNSON.—THE PRACTICAL DRAUGHTSMAN'S BOOK OF INDUSTRIAL DESIGN, AND MACHINIST'S AND ENGINEER'S DRAWING COMPANION: Forming a complete course of Mechanical Engineering and Architectural Drawing. From the French of M. Armengaud the elder, Prof. of Design in the Conservatoire of Arts and Industry, Paris, and MM. Armengaud the younger and Amouroux, Civil Engineers. Rewritten and arranged, with additional matter and plates, selections from and examples of the most useful and generally employed mechanism of the day. By William Johnson, Assoc. Inst. C. E., Editor of "The Practical Mechanic's Journal." Illustrated by 50 folio steel plates and 50 wood-cuts. A new edition, 4to. . $10 00

ARLOT.—A COMPLETE GUIDE FOR COACH PAINTERS. Translated from the French of M. Arlot, Coach Painter; late Master Painter for eleven years with M. Ehrler, Coach Manufacturer, Paris. With important American additions . . $1 25

ARROWSMITH.—PAPER-HANGER'S COMPANION: A Treatise in which the Practical Operations of the Trade are Systematically laid down: with Copious Directions Preparatory to Papering; Preventives against the Effect of Damp on Walls; the Various Cements and Pastes adapted to the Several Purposes of the Trade; Observations and Directions for the Panelling and Ornamenting of Rooms, &c. By James Arrowsmith. 12mo., cloth $1 25

BAIRD.—THE AMERICAN COTTON SPINNER, AND MANAGER'S AND CARDER'S GUIDE:

A Practical Treatise on Cotton Spinning; giving the Dimensions and Speed of Machinery, Draught and Twist Calculations, etc.; with notices of recent Improvements: together with Rules and Examples for making changes in the sizes and numbers of Roving and Yarn. Compiled from the papers of the late ROBERT H. BAIRD. 12mo. $1 50

BAKER.—LONG-SPAN RAILWAY BRIDGES:

Comprising Investigations of the Comparative Theoretical and Practical Advantages of the various Adopted or Proposed Type Systems of Construction; with numerous Formulæ and Tables. By B. Baker. 12mo. $2 00

BAKEWELL.—A MANUAL OF ELECTRICITY—PRACTICAL AND THEORETICAL:

By F. C. BAKEWELL, Inventor of the Copying Telegraph. Second Edition. Revised and enlarged. Illustrated by numerous engravings. 12mo. Cloth $2 00

BEANS.—A TREATISE ON RAILROAD CURVES AND THE LOCATION OF RAILROADS:

By E. W. BEANS, C. E. 12mo. (In press.)

BLENKARN.—PRACTICAL SPECIFICATIONS OF WORKS EXECUTED IN ARCHITECTURE, CIVIL AND MECHANICAL ENGINEERING, AND IN ROAD MAKING AND SEWERING:

To which are added a series of practically useful Agreements and Reports. By JOHN BLENKARN. Illustrated by fifteen large folding plates. 8vo. $9 00

BLINN.—A PRACTICAL WORKSHOP COMPANION FOR TIN, SHEET-IRON, AND COPPER-PLATE WORKERS:

Containing Rules for Describing various kinds of Patterns used by Tin, Sheet-iron, and Copper-plate Workers; Practical Geometry; Mensuration of Surfaces and Solids; Tables of the Weight of Metals, Lead Pipe, etc.; Tables of Areas and Circumferences of Circles; Japans, Varnishes, Lackers, Cements, Compositions, etc. etc. By LEROY J. BLINN, Master Mechanic. With over One Hundred Illustrations. 12mo. $2 50

BOOTH.—MARBLE WORKER'S MANUAL:
Containing Practical Information respecting Marbles in general, their Cutting, Working, and Polishing; Veneering of Marble; Mosaics; Composition and Use of Artificial Marble, Stuccos, Cements, Receipts, Secrets, etc. etc. Translated from the French by M. L. BOOTH. With an Appendix concerning American Marbles. 12mo., cloth . . $1 50

BOOTH AND MORFIT.—THE ENCYCLOPEDIA OF CHEMISTRY, PRACTICAL AND THEORETICAL:
Embracing its application to the Arts, Metallurgy, Mineralogy, Geology, Medicine, and Pharmacy. By JAMES C. BOOTH, Melter and Refiner in the United States Mint, Professor of Applied Chemistry in the Franklin Institute, etc., assisted by CAMPBELL MORFIT, author of "Chemical Manipulations," etc. Seventh edition. Complete in one volume, royal 8vo., 978 pages, with numerous wood-cuts and other illustrations. $5 00

BOWDITCH.—ANALYSIS, TECHNICAL VALUATION, PURIFICATION, AND USE OF COAL GAS:
By Rev. W. R. BOWDITCH. Illustrated with wood engravings. 8vo. $6 50

BOX.—PRACTICAL HYDRAULICS:
A Series of Rules and Tables for the use of Engineers, etc. By THOMAS BOX. 12mo. $2 00

BUCKMASTER.—THE ELEMENTS OF MECHANICAL PHYSICS:
By J. C. BUCKMASTER, late Student in the Government School of Mines; Certified Teacher of Science by the Department of Science and Art; Examiner in Chemistry and Physics in the Royal College of Preceptors; and late Lecturer in Chemistry and Physics of the Royal Polytechnic Institute. Illustrated with numerous engravings. In one vol. 12mo. . $1 50

BULLOCK.—THE AMERICAN COTTAGE BUILDER:
A Series of Designs, Plans, and Specifications, from $200 to to $20,000 for Homes for the People; together with Warming, Ventilation, Drainage, Painting, and Landscape Gardening. By JOHN BULLOCK, Architect, Civil Engineer, Mechanician, and Editor of "The Rudiments of Architecture and Building," etc. Illustrated by 75 engravings. In one vol. 8vo. $3 50

BULLOCK.—THE RUDIMENTS OF ARCHITECTURE AND BUILDING:

For the use of Architects, Builders, Draughtsmen, Machinists, Engineers, and Mechanics. Edited by JOHN BULLOCK, author of "The American Cottage Builder." Illustrated by 250 engravings. In one volume 8vo. . . . $3 50

BURGH.—PRACTICAL ILLUSTRATIONS OF LAND AND MARINE ENGINES:

Showing in detail the Modern Improvements of High and Low Pressure, Surface Condensation, and Super-heating, together with Land and Marine Boilers. By N. P. BURGH, Engineer. Illustrated by twenty plates, double elephant folio, with text. $21 00

BURGH.—PRACTICAL RULES FOR THE PROPORTIONS OF MODERN ENGINES AND BOILERS FOR LAND AND MARINE PURPOSES.

By N. P. BURGH, Engineer. 12mo. . . . $2 00

BURGH.—THE SLIDE-VALVE PRACTICALLY CONSIDERED:

By N. P. BURGH, author of "A Treatise on Sugar Machinery," "Practical Illustrations of Land and Marine Engines," "A Pocket-Book of Practical Rules for Designing Land and Marine Engines, Boilers," etc. etc. etc. Completely illustrated. 12mo. $2 00

BYRN.—THE COMPLETE PRACTICAL BREWER:

Or, Plain, Accurate, and Thorough Instructions in the Art of Brewing Beer, Ale, Porter, including the Process of making Bavarian Beer, all the Small Beers, such as Root-beer, Ginger-pop, Sarsaparilla-beer, Mead, Spruce beer, etc. etc. Adapted to the use of Public Brewers and Private Families. By M. LA FAYETTE BYRN, M. D. With illustrations. 12mo. $1 25

BYRN.—THE COMPLETE PRACTICAL DISTILLER:

Comprising the most perfect and exact Theoretical and Practical Description of the Art of Distillation and Rectification; including all of the most recent improvements in distilling apparatus; instructions for preparing spirits from the numerous vegetables, fruits, etc.; directions for the distillation and preparation of all kinds of brandies and other spirits, spirituous and other compounds, etc. etc.; all of which is so simplified that it is adapted not only to the use of extensive distillers, but for every farmer, or others who may wish to engage in the art of distilling By M. LA FAYETTE BYRN, M. D. With numerous engravings. In one volume, 12mo. $1 50

BYRNE.—POCKET BOOK FOR RAILROAD AND CIVIL ENGINEERS:
Containing New, Exact, and Concise Methods for Laying out Railroad Curves, Switches, Frog Angles and Crossings; the Staking out of work; Levelling; the Calculation of Cuttings; Embankments; Earth-work, etc. By OLIVER BYRNE. Illustrated, 18mo., full bound $1 75

BYRNE.—THE HANDBOOK FOR THE ARTISAN, MECHANIC, AND ENGINEER:
By OLIVER BYRNE. Illustrated by 185 Wood Engravings. 8vo. $5 00

BYRNE.—THE ESSENTIAL ELEMENTS OF PRACTICAL MECHANICS:
For Engineering Students, based on the Principle of Work. By OLIVER BYRNE. Illustrated by Numerous Wood Engravings, 12mo. $3 63

BYRNE.—THE PRACTICAL METAL-WORKER'S ASSISTANT:
Comprising Metallurgic Chemistry; the Arts of Working all Metals and Alloys; Forging of Iron and Steel; Hardening and Tempering; Melting and Mixing; Casting and Founding; Works in Sheet Metal; the Processes Dependent on the Ductility of the Metals; Soldering; and the most Improved Processes and Tools employed by Metal-Workers. With the Application of the Art of Electro-Metallurgy to Manufacturing Processes; collected from Original Sources, and from the Works of Holtzapffel, Bergeron, Leupold, Plumier, Napier, and others. By OLIVER BYRNE. A New, Revised, and improved Edition, with Additions by John Scoffern, M. B , William Clay, Wm. Fairbairn, F. R. S., and James Napier. With Five Hundred and Ninety-two Engravings; Illustrating every Branch of the Subject. In one volume, 8vo. 652 pages . $7 00

BYRNE.—THE PRACTICAL MODEL CALCULATOR:
For the Engineer, Mechanic, Manufacturer of Engine Work, Naval Architect, Miner, and Millwright. By OLIVER BYRNE. 1 volume, 8vo., nearly 600 pages $4 50

BEMROSE.—MANUAL OF WOOD CARVING: With Practical Illustrations for Learners of the Art, and Original and Selected designs. By WILLIAM BEMROSE, Jr. With an Introduction by LLEWELLYN JEWITT, F. S. A., etc. With 128 Illustrations. 4to., cloth $3 00

BAIRD.—PROTECTION OF HOME LABOR AND HOME PRODUCTIONS NECESSARY TO THE PROSPERITY OF THE AMERICAN FARMER:

By HENRY CAREY BAIRD. 8vo., paper 10

BAIRD.—THE RIGHTS OF AMERICAN PRODUCERS, AND THE WRONGS OF BRITISH FREE TRADE REVENUE REFORM.

By HENRY CAREY BAIRD. (1870) 5

BAIRD.—SOME OF THE FALLACIES OF BRITISH-FREE-TRADE REVENUE-REFORM.

Two Letters to Prof. A. L. Perry, of Williams College, Mass. By HENRY CAREY BAIRD. (1871.) Paper 5

BAIRD.—STANDARD WAGES COMPUTING TABLES:

An Improvement in all former Methods of Computation, so arranged that wages for days, hours, or fractions of hours, at a specified rate per day or hour, may be ascertained at a glance. By T. SPANGLER BAIRD. Oblong folio $5 00

BAUERMAN.—TREATISE ON THE METALLURGY OF IRON.

Illustrated. 12mo. $2 50

BICKNELL'S VILLAGE BUILDER.

55 large plates. 4to. $10 00

BISHOP.—A HISTORY OF AMERICAN MANUFACTURES:

From 1608 to 1866; exhibiting the Origin and Growth of the Principal Mechanic Arts and Manufactures, from the Earliest Colonial Period to the Present Time; By J. LEANDER BISHOP, M. D., EDWARD YOUNG, and EDWIN T. FREEDLEY. Three vols. 8vo., half morocco $12 00

BOX.—A PRACTICAL TREATISE ON HEAT AS APPLIED TO THE USEFUL ARTS:

For the use of Engineers, Architects, etc. By THOMAS BOX, author of "Practical Hydraulics." Illustrated by 14 plates, containing 114 figures. 12mo. $4 25

CABINET MAKER'S ALBUM OF FURNITURE:

Comprising a Collection of Designs for the Newest and Most Elegant Styles of Furniture. Illustrated by Forty-eight Large and Beautifully Engraved Plates. In one volume, oblong $5 00

CHAPMAN.—A TREATISE ON ROPE-MAKING:

As practised in private and public Rope-yards, with a Description of the Manufacture, Rules, Tables of Weights, etc., adapted to the Trade; Shipping, Mining, Railways, Builders, etc. By ROBERT CHAPMAN. 24mo. $1 50

CRAIK.—THE PRACTICAL AMERICAN MILLWRIGHT AND MILLER.

Comprising the Elementary Principles of Mechanics, Mechanism, and Motive Power, Hydraulics and Hydraulic Motors, Mill-dams, Saw Mills, Grist Mills, the Oat Meal Mill, the Barley Mill, Wool Carding, and Cloth Fulling and Dressing, Wind Mills, Steam Power, &c. By DAVID CRAIK, Millwright. Illustrated by numerous wood engravings, and five folding plates. 1 vol. 8vo. $5 00

CAMPIN.—A PRACTICAL TREATISE ON MECHANICAL ENGINEERING:

Comprising Metallurgy, Moulding, Casting, Forging, Tools, Workshop Machinery, Mechanical Manipulation, Manufacture of Steam-engines, etc. etc. With an Appendix on the Analysis of Iron and Iron Ores. By FRANCIS CAMPIN, C. E. To which are added, Observations on the Construction of Steam Boilers, and Remarks upon Furnaces used for Smoke Prevention; with a Chapter on Explosions. By R. Armstrong, C. E., and John Bourne. Rules for Calculating the Change Wheels for Screws on a Turning Lathe, and for a Wheel-cutting Machine. By J. LA NICCA. Management of Steel, including Forging, Hardening, Tempering, Annealing, Shrinking, and Expansion. And the Case-hardening of Iron. By G. EDE. 8vo. Illustrated with 29 plates and 100 wood engravings.

$6 00

CAMPIN.—THE PRACTICE OF HAND-TURNING IN WOOD, IVORY, SHELL, ETC.:

With Instructions for Turning such works in Metal as may be required in the Practice of Turning Wood, Ivory, etc. Also, an Appendix on Ornamental Turning. By FRANCIS CAMPIN, with Numerous Illustrations, 12mo., cloth . . . $3 00

CAPRON DE DOLE.—DUSSAUCE.—BLUES AND CARMINES OF INDIGO.

A Practical Treatise on the Fabrication of every Commercial Product derived from Indigo. By FELICIEN CAPRON DE DOLE. Translated, with important additions, by Professor H. DUSSAUCE. 12mo. $2 50

CAREY.—THE WORKS OF HENRY C. CAREY:

CONTRACTION OR EXPANSION? REPUDIATION OR RESUMPTION? Letters to Hon. Hugh McCulloch. 8vo. 38

FINANCIAL CRISES, their Causes and Effects. 8vo. paper 25

HARMONY OF INTERESTS; Agricultural, Manufacturing, and Commercial. 8vo., paper $1 00
Do. do. cloth $1 50

LETTERS TO THE PRESIDENT OF THE UNITED STATES. Paper $1 00

MANUAL OF SOCIAL SCIENCE. Condensed from Carey's "Principles of Social Science." By KATE MCKEAN. 1 vol. 12mo. $2 25

MISCELLANEOUS WORKS: comprising "Harmony of Interests," "Money," "Letters to the President," "French and American Tariffs," "Financial Crises," "The Way to Outdo England without Fighting Her," "Resources of the Union," "The Public Debt," "Contraction or Expansion," "Review of the Decade 1857—'67," "Reconstruction," etc. etc. 1 vol. 8vo., cloth $4 50

MONEY: A LECTURE before the N. Y. Geographical and Statistical Society. 8vo., paper 25

PAST, PRESENT, AND FUTURE. 8vo. $2 50

PRINCIPLES OF SOCIAL SCIENCE. 3 volumes 8vo., cloth $10 00

REVIEW OF THE DECADE 1857—'67. 8vo., paper 50

RECONSTRUCTION: INDUSTRIAL, FINANCIAL, AND POLITICAL. Letters to the Hon. Henry Wilson, U. S. S. 8vo, paper 50

THE PUBLIC DEBT, LOCAL AND NATIONAL. How to provide for its discharge while lessening the burden of Taxation. Letter to David A. Wells, Esq., U. S. Revenue Commission. 8vo., paper 25

THE RESOURCES OF THE UNION. A Lecture read, Dec. 1865, before the American Geographical and Statistical Society, N. Y., and before the American Association for the Advancement of Social Science, Boston 50

THE SLAVE TRADE, DOMESTIC AND FOREIGN; Why it Exists, and How it may be Extinguished. 12mo., cloth $1 50

LETTERS ON INTERNATIONAL COPYRIGHT. (1867.) Paper 50

REVIEW OF THE FARMERS' QUESTION. (1870.) Paper 25

RESUMPTION! HOW IT MAY PROFITABLY BE BROUGHT AROUT. (1869.) 8vo., paper 50

REVIEW OF THE REPORT OF HON. D. A. WELLS, Special Commissioner of the Revenue. (1869.) 8vo., paper 50

SHALL WE HAVE PEACE? Peace Financial and Peace Political. Letters to the President Elect. (1868.) 8vo., paper 50

THE FINANCE MINISTER AND THE CURRENCY, AND THE PUBLIC DEBT. (1868.) 8vo., paper . . 50

THE WAY TO OUTDO ENGLAND WITHOUT FIGHTING HER. Letters to Hon. Schuyler Colfax. (1865.) 8vo., paper $1 00

WEALTH! OF WHAT DOES IT CONSIST? (1870.) Paper 25

CAMUS.—A TREATISE ON THE TEETH OF WHEELS:

Demonstrating the best forms which can be given to them for the purposes of Machinery, such as Mill-work and Clock-work. Translated from the French of M. CAMUS. By JOHN I. HAWKINS. Illustrated by 40 plates. 8vo. $3 00

COXE.—MINING LEGISLATION.

A paper read before the Am. Social Science Association. By ECKLEY B. COXE. Paper 20

COLBURN.—THE GAS-WORKS OF LONDON:

Comprising a sketch of the Gas-works of the city, Process of Manufacture, Quantity Produced, Cost, Profit, etc. By ZERAH COLBURN. 8vo., cloth 75

COLBURN.—THE LOCOMOTIVE ENGINE:

Including a Description of its Structure, Rules for Estimating its Capabilities, and Practical Observations on its Construction and Management. By ZERAH COLBURN. Illustrated. A new edition. 12mo. $1 25

COLBURN AND MAW.—THE WATER-WORKS OF LONDON:

Together with a Series of Articles on various other Waterworks. By ZERAH COLBURN and W. MAW. Reprinted from "Engineering." In one volume, 8vo. . . $4 00

DAGUERREOTYPIST AND PHOTOGRAPHER'S COMPANION:

12mo., cloth $1 25

DIRCKS.—PERPETUAL MOTION:

Or Search for Self-Motive Power during the 17th, 18th, and 19th centuries. Illustrated from various authentic sources in Papers, Essays, Letters, Paragraphs, and numerous Patent Specifications, with an Introductory Essay by HENRY DIRCKS, C. E. Illustrated by numerous engravings of machines. 12mo., cloth $3 50

DIXON.—THE PRACTICAL MILLWRIGHT'S AND ENGINEER'S GUIDE:

Or Tables for Finding the Diameter and Power of Cogwheels; Diameter, Weight, and Power of Shafts; Diameter and Strength of Bolts, etc. etc. By THOMAS DIXON. 12mo., cloth. $1 50

DUNCAN.—PRACTICAL SURVEYOR'S GUIDE:

Containing the necessary information to make any person, of common capacity, a finished land surveyor without the aid of a teacher. By ANDREW DUNCAN. Illustrated. 12mo., cloth. $1 25

DUSSAUCE.—A NEW AND COMPLETE TREATISE ON THE ARTS OF TANNING, CURRYING, AND LEATHER DRESSING:

Comprising all the Discoveries and Improvements made in France, Great Britain, and the United States. Edited from Notes and Documents of Messrs. Sallerou, Grouvelle, Duval, Dessables, Labarraque, Payen, René, De Fontenelle, Malapeyre, etc. etc. By Prof. H. DUSSAUCE, Chemist. Illustrated by 212 wood engravings. 8vo. $10 00

DUSSAUCE.—A GENERAL TREATISE ON THE MANUFACTURE OF SOAP, THEORETICAL AND PRACTICAL:

Comprising the Chemistry of the Art, a Description of all the Raw Materials and their Uses. Directions for the Establishment of a Soap Factory, with the necessary Apparatus, Instructions in the Manufacture of every variety of Soap, the Assay and Determination of the Value of Alkalies, Fatty Substances, Soaps, etc. etc. By PROFESSOR H. DUSSAUCE. With an Appendix, containing Extracts from the Reports of the International Jury on Soaps, as exhibited in the Paris Universal Exposition, 1867, numerous Tables, etc. etc. Illustrated by engravings. In one volume 8vo. of over 800 pages $10 00

DUSSAUCE.—PRACTICAL TREATISE ON THE FABRICATION OF MATCHES, GUN COTTON, AND FULMINATING POWDERS.

By Professor H. DUSSAUCE. 12mo. . . . $3 00

DUSSAUCE.—A PRACTICAL GUIDE FOR THE PERFUMER:
Being a New Treatise on Perfumery the most favorable to the Beauty without being injurious to the Health, comprising a Description of the substances used in Perfumery, the Formulæ of more than one thousand Preparations, such as Cosmetics, Perfumed Oils, Tooth Powders, Waters, Extracts, Tinctures, Infusions, Vinaigres, Essential Oils, Pastels, Creams, Soaps, and many new Hygienic Products not hitherto described. Edited from Notes and Documents of Messrs. Debay, Lunel, etc. With additions by Professor H. DUSSAUCE, Chemist. 12mo. $3 00

DUSSAUCE.—A GENERAL TREATISE ON THE MANUFACTURE OF VINEGAR, THEORETICAL AND PRACTICAL.
Comprising the various methods, by the slow and the quick processes, with Alcohol, Wine, Grain, Cider, and Molasses, as well as the Fabrication of Wood Vinegar, etc. By Prof. H. DUSSAUCE. 12mo. (*In press.*)

DUPLAIS.—A COMPLETE TREATISE ON THE DISTILLATION AND MANUFACTURE OF ALCOHOLIC LIQUORS:
From the French of M. DUPLAIS. Translated and Edited by M. MCKENNIE, M D. Illustrated by numerous large plates and wood engravings of the best apparatus calculated for producing the finest products. In one vol. royal 8vo. (Ready May 1, 1871.)

☞ This is a treatise of the highest scientific merit and of the greatest practical value, surpassing in these respects, as well as in the variety of its contents, any similar volume in the English language.

DE GRAFF.—THE GEOMETRICAL STAIR-BUILDERS' GUIDE:
Being a Plain Practical System of Hand-Railing, embracing all its necessary Details, and Geometrically Illustrated by 22 Steel Engravings; together with the use of the most approved principles of Practical Geometry. By SIMON DE GRAFF, Architect. 4to. $5 00

DYER AND COLOR-MAKER'S COMPANION:
Containing upwards of two hundred Receipts for making Colors, on the most approved principles, for all the various styles and fabrics now in existence; with the Scouring Process, and plain Directions for Preparing, Washing-off, and Finishing the Goods. In one vol. 12mo. $1 25

EASTON.—A PRACTICAL TREATISE ON STREET OR HORSE-POWER RAILWAYS:

Their Location, Construction, and Management; with General Plans and Rules for their Organization and Operation; together with Examinations as to their Comparative Advantages over the Omnibus System, and Inquiries as to their Value for Investment; including Copies of Municipal Ordinances relating thereto. By ALEXANDER EASTON, C. E. Illustrated by 23 plates, 8vo., cloth $2 00

FORSYTH.—BOOK OF DESIGNS FOR HEAD-STONES, MURAL, AND OTHER MONUMENTS:

Containing 78 Elaborate and Exquisite Designs. By FORSYTH. 4to., cloth $5 00

*** This volume, for the beauty and variety of its designs, has never been surpassed by any publication of the kind, and should be in the hands of every marble-worker who does fine monumental work.

FAIRBAIRN.—THE PRINCIPLES OF MECHANISM AND MACHINERY OF TRANSMISSION:

Comprising the Principles of Mechanism, Wheels, and Pulleys, Strength and Proportions of Shafts, Couplings of Shafts, and Engaging and Disengaging Gear. By WILLIAM FAIRBAIRN, Esq., C. E., LL. D., F. R. S., F. G. S., Corresponding Member of the National Institute of France, and of the Royal Academy of Turin; Chevalier of the Legion of Honor, etc. etc. Beautifully illustrated by over 150 wood-cuts. In one volume 12mo. $2 50

FAIRBAIRN.—PRIME-MOVERS:

Comprising the Accumulation of Water-power; the Construction of Water-wheels and Turbines; the Properties of Steam; the Varieties of Steam-engines and Boilers and Wind-mills. By WILLIAM FAIRBAIRN, C. E., LL. D., F. R. S., F. G. S. Author of "Principles of Mechanism and the Machinery of Transmission." With Numerous Illustrations. In one volume. (In press.)

GILBART.—A PRACTICAL TREATISE ON BANKING:

By JAMES WILLIAM GILBART. To which is added: THE NATIONAL BANK ACT AS NOW IN FORCE. 8vo. . . . $4 50

GESNER.—A PRACTICAL TREATISE ON COAL, PETROLEUM, AND OTHER DISTILLED OILS.

By ABRAHAM GESNER, M. D., F. G. S. Second edition, revised and enlarged. By GEORGE WELTDEN GESNER, Consulting Chemist and Engineer. Illustrated. 8vo. . . . $3 50

GOTHIC ALBUM FOR CABINET MAKERS:

Comprising a Collection of Designs for Gothic Furniture. Illustrated by twenty-three large and beautifully engraved plates. Oblong $3 00

GRANT.—BEET-ROOT SUGAR AND CULTIVATION OF THE BEET:

By E. B. GRANT. 12mo. $1 25

GREGORY.—MATHEMATICS FOR PRACTICAL MEN:

Adapted to the Pursuits of Surveyors, Architects, Mechanics, and Civil Engineers. By OLINTHUS GREGORY. 8vo., plates, cloth $3 00

GRISWOLD.—RAILROAD ENGINEER'S POCKET COMPANION.

Comprising Rules for Calculating Deflection Distances and Angles, Tangential Distances and Angles, and all Necessary Tables for Engineers; also the art of Levelling from Preliminary Survey to the Construction of Railroads, intended Expressly for the Young Engineer, together with Numerous Valuable Rules and Examples. By W. GRISWOLD. 12mo., tucks. $1 75

GUETTIER.—METALLIC ALLOYS:

Being a Practical Guide to their Chemical and Physical Properties, their Preparation, Composition, and Uses. Translated from the French of A. GUETTIER, Engineer and Director of Founderies, author of "La Fouderie en France," etc. etc. By A. A. FESQUET, Chemist and Engineer. In one volume, 12mo. (In press.)

HATS AND FELTING:

A Practical Treatise on their Manufacture. By a Practical Hatter. Illustrated by Drawings of Machinery, &c., 8vo. $1 25

HAY.—THE INTERIOR DECORATOR:

The Laws of Harmonious Coloring adapted to Interior Decorations: with a Practical Treatise on House-Painting. By D. R. HAY, House-Painter and Decorator. Illustrated by a Diagram of the Primary, Secondary, and Tertiary Colors. 12mo. $2 25

HUGHES.—AMERICAN MILLER AND MILLWRIGHT'S ASSISTANT:

By WM. CARTER HUGHES. A new edition. In one volume, 12mo. $1 50

HUNT.—THE PRACTICE OF PHOTOGRAPHY.

By ROBERT HUNT, Vice-President of the Photographic Society, London. With numerous illustrations. 12mo., cloth . 75

HURST.—A HAND-BOOK FOR ARCHITECTURAL SURVEYORS:

Comprising Formulæ useful in Designing Builders' work, Table of Weights, of the materials used in Building, Memoranda connected with Builders' work, Mensuration, the Practice of Builders' Measurement, Contracts of Labor, Valuation of Property, Summary of the Practice in Dilapidation, etc. etc. By J. F. HURST, C. E. 2d edition, pocket-book form, full bound $2 50

JERVIS.—RAILWAY PROPERTY:

A Treatise on the Construction and Management of Railways; designed to afford useful knowledge, in the popular style, to the holders of this class of property; as well as Railway Managers, Officers, and Agents. By JOHN B. JERVIS, late Chief Engineer of the Hudson River Railroad, Croton Aqueduct, &c. One vol. 12mo., cloth $2 00

JOHNSON.—A REPORT TO THE NAVY DEPARTMENT OF THE UNITED STATES ON AMERICAN COALS:

Applicable to Steam Navigation and to other purposes. By WALTER R. JOHNSON. With numerous illustrations. 607 pp. 8vo., half morocco $10 00

JOHNSTON.—INSTRUCTIONS FOR THE ANALYSIS OF SOILS, LIMESTONES, AND MANURES.

By J. W. F. JOHNSTON. 12mo. 35

KEENE.—A HAND-BOOK OF PRACTICAL GAUGING,

For the Use of Beginners, to which is added a Chapter on Distillation, describing the process in operation at the Custom House for ascertaining the strength of wines. By JAMES B. KEENE, of H. M. Customs. 8vo. . . . $1 25

KENTISH.—A TREATISE ON A BOX OF INSTRUMENTS,

And the Slide Rule; with the Theory of Trigonometry and Logarithms, including Practical Geometry, Surveying, Measuring of Timber, Cask and Malt Gauging, Heights, and Distances. By THOMAS KENTISH. In one volume. 12mo. . . $1 25

KOBELL.—ERNI.—MINERALOGY SIMPLIFIED:

A short method of Determining and Classifying Minerals, by means of simple Chemical Experiments in the Wet Way. Translated from the last German Edition of F. VON KOBELL, with an Introduction to Blowpipe Analysis and other additions. By HENRI ERNI, M. D., Chief Chemist, Department of Agriculture, author of "Coal Oil and Petroleum." In one volume. 12mo. $2 50

LANDRIN.—A TREATISE ON STEEL:

Comprising its Theory, Metallurgy, Properties, Practical Working, and Use. By M. H. C. LANDRIN, Jr., Civil Engineer. Translated from the French, with Notes, by A. A. FESQUET, Chemist and Engineer. With an Appendix on the Bessemer and the Martin Processes for Manufacturing Steel, from the Report of ABRAM S. HEWITT, United States Commissioner to the Universal Exposition, Paris, 1867. 12mo. . . $3 00

LARKIN.—THE PRACTICAL BRASS AND IRON FOUNDER'S GUIDE.

A Concise Treatise on Brass Founding, Moulding, the Metals and their Alloys, etc.; to which are added Recent Improvements in the Manufacture of Iron, Steel by the Bessemer Process, etc. etc. By JAMES LARKIN, late Conductor of the Brass Foundry Department in Reany, Neafie & Co.'s Penn Works, Philadelphia. Fifth edition, revised, with extensive Additions. In one volume. 12mo. $2 25

LEAVITT.—FACTS ABOUT PEAT AS AN ARTICLE OF FUEL:

With Remarks upon its Origin and Composition, the Localities in which it is found, the Methods of Preparation and Manufacture, and the various Uses to which it is applicable; together with many other matters of Practical and Scientific Interest. To which is added a chapter on the Utilization of Coal Dust with Peat for the Production of an Excellent Fuel at Moderate Cost, especially adapted for Steam Service. By H. T. LEAVITT. Third edition. 12mo. $1 75

LEROUX.—A PRACTICAL TREATISE ON THE MANUFACTURE OF WORSTEDS AND CARDED YARNS:

Translated from the French of CHARLES LEROUX, Mechanical Engineer, and Superintendent of a Spinning Mill. By Dr. H. PAINE, and A. A. FESQUET. Illustrated by 12 large plates. In one volume 8vo. $5 00

LESLIE (MISS).—COMPLETE COOKERY:

Directions for Cookery in its Various Branches. By MISS LESLIE. 60th edition. Thoroughly revised, with the addition of New Receipts. In 1 vol. 12mo., cloth . . $1 50

LESLIE (MISS). LADIES' HOUSE BOOK:

a Manual of Domestic Economy. 20th revised edition. 12mo., cloth $1 25

LESLIE (MISS).—TWO HUNDRED RECEIPTS IN FRENCH COOKERY.

12mo. 50

LIEBER.—ASSAYER'S GUIDE:

Or, Practical Directions to Assayers, Miners, and Smelters, for the Tests and Assays, by Heat and by Wet Processes, for the Ores of all the principal Metals, of Gold and Silver Coins and Alloys, and of Coal, etc. By OSCAR M. LIEBER. 12mo., cloth $1 25

LOVE.—THE ART OF DYEING, CLEANING, SCOURING, AND FINISHING:

On the most approved English and French methods; being Practical Instructions in Dyeing Silks, Woollens, and Cottons, Feathers, Chips, Straw, etc.; Scouring and Cleaning Bed and Window Curtains, Carpets, Rugs, etc.; French and English Cleaning, etc. By THOMAS LOVE. Second American Edition, to which are added General Instructions for the Use of Aniline Colors. 8vo. 5 00

MAIN AND BROWN.—QUESTIONS ON SUBJECTS CONNECTED WITH THE MARINE STEAM-ENGINE:

And Examination Papers; with Hints for their Solution. By THOMAS J. MAIN, Professor of Mathematics, Royal Naval College, and THOMAS BROWN, Chief Engineer, R. N. 12mo., cloth $1 50

MAIN AND BROWN.—THE INDICATOR AND DYNAMOMETER:

With their Practical Applications to the Steam-Engine. By THOMAS J. MAIN, M. A. F. R., Ass't Prof. Royal Naval College, Portsmouth, and THOMAS BROWN, Assoc. Inst. C. E., Chief Engineer, R. N., attached to the R. N. College. Illustrated. From the Fourth London Edition. 8vo. $1 50

MAIN AND BROWN.—THE MARINE STEAM-ENGINE.

By THOMAS J. MAIN, F. R. Ass't S. Mathematical Professor at Royal Naval College, and THOMAS BROWN, Assoc. Inst. C. E. Chief Engineer, R. N. Attached to the Royal Naval College. Authors of "Questions Connected with the Marine Steam-Engine," and the "Indicator and Dynamometer." With numerous Illustrations. In one volume 8vo. $5 00

MARTIN.—SCREW-CUTTING TABLES, FOR THE USE OF MECHANICAL ENGINEERS:

Showing the Proper Arrangement of Wheels for Cutting the Threads of Screws of any required Pitch; with a Table for Making the Universal Gas-Pipe Thread and Taps. By W. A. MARTIN, Engineer. 8vo. 50

MILES—A PLAIN TREATISE ON HORSE-SHOEING.

With Illustrations. By WILLIAM MILES, author of "The Horse's Foot" $1 00

MOLESWORTH.—POCKET-BOOK OF USEFUL FORMULÆ AND MEMORANDA FOR CIVIL AND MECHANICAL ENGINEERS.

By GUILFORD L. MOLESWORTH, Member of the Institution of Civil Engineers, Chief Resident Engineer of the Ceylon Railway. Second American from the Tenth London Edition. In one volume, full bound in pocket-book form $2 00

MOORE.—THE INVENTOR'S GUIDE:

Patent Office and Patent Laws: or, a Guide to Inventors, and a Book of Reference for Judges, Lawyers, Magistrates, and others. By J. G. MOORE. 12mo., cloth $1 25

NAPIER.—A MANUAL OF ELECTRO-METALLURGY:

Including the Application of the Art to Manufacturing Processes. By JAMES NAPIER. Fourth American, from the Fourth London edition, revised and enlarged. Illustrated by engravings. In one volume, 8vo. $2 00

NAPIER.—A SYSTEM OF CHEMISTRY APPLIED TO DYEING:
By JAMES NAPIER, F. C. S. A New and Thoroughly Revised Edition, completely brought up to the present state of the Science, including the Chemistry of Coal Tar Colors. By A. A. FESQUET, Chemist and Engineer. With an Appendix on Dyeing and Calico Printing, as shown at the Paris Universal Exposition of 1867, from the Reports of the International Jury, etc. Illustrated. In one volume 8vo., 400 pages $5 00

NEWBERY.—GLEANINGS FROM ORNAMENTAL ART OF EVERY STYLE;
Drawn from Examples in the British, South Kensington, Indian, Crystal Palace, and other Museums, the Exhibitions of 1851 and 1862, and the best English and Foreign works. In a series of one hundred exquisitely drawn Plates, containing many hundred examples. By ROBERT NEWBERY. 4to. $15 00

NICHOLSON.—A MANUAL OF THE ART OF BOOK-BINDING:
Containing full instructions in the different Branches of Forwarding, Gilding, and Finishing. Also, the Art of Marbling Book-edges and Paper. By JAMES B. NICHOLSON. Illustrated. 12mo. cloth $2 25

NORRIS.—A HAND-BOOK FOR LOCOMOTIVE ENGINEERS AND MACHINISTS:
Comprising the Proportions and Calculations for Constructing Locomotives; Manner of Setting Valves; Tables of Squares, Cubes, Areas, etc. etc. By SEPTIMUS NORRIS, Civil and Mechanical Engineer. New edition. Illustrated, 12mo., cloth $2 00

NYSTROM.—ON TECHNOLOGICAL EDUCATION AND THE CONSTRUCTION OF SHIPS AND SCREW PROPELLERS:
For Naval and Marine Engineers. By JOHN W. NYSTROM, late Acting Chief Engineer U. S. N. Second edition, revised with additional matter. Illustrated by seven engravings. 12mo. $2 50

O'NEILL.—A DICTIONARY OF DYEING AND CALICO PRINTING:
Containing a brief account of all the Substances and Processes in use in the Art of Dyeing and Printing Textile Fabrics: with Practical Receipts and Scientific Information. By CHARLES O'NEILL, Analytical Chemist; Fellow of the Chemical Society of London; Member of the Literary and Philosophical Society of Manchester; Author of "Chemistry of Calico Printing and Dyeing." To which is added An Essay on Coal Tar Colors and their Application to

Dyeing and Calico Printing. By A. A. FESQUET, Chemist and Engineer. With an Appendix on Dyeing and Calico Printing, as shown at the Exposition of 1867, from the Reports of the International Jury, etc. In one volume 8vo., 491 pages . . $6 00

OSBORN.—THE METALLURGY OF IRON AND STEEL:

Theoretical and Practical: In all its Branches; With Special Reference to American Materials and Processes. By H. S. OSBORN, LL. D., Professor of Mining and Metallurgy in Lafayette College, Easton, Pa. Illustrated by 230 Engravings on Wood, and 6 Folding Plates. 8vo., 972 pages $10 00

OSBORN.—AMERICAN MINES AND MINING:

Theoretically and Practically Considered. By Prof. H. S. OSBORN, Illustrated by numerous engravings. 8vo. (*In preparation.*)

PAINTER, GILDER, AND VARNISHER'S COMPANION:

Containing Rules and Regulations in everything relating to the Arts of Painting, Gilding, Varnishing, and Glass Staining, with numerous useful and valuable Receipts; Tests for the Detection of Adulterations in Oils and Colors, and a statement of the Diseases and Accidents to which Painters, Gilders, and Varnishers are particularly liable, with the simplest methods of Prevention and Remedy. With Directions for Graining, Marbling, Sign Writing, and Gilding on Glass. To which are added COMPLETE INSTRUCTIONS FOR COACH PAINTING AND VARNISHING. 12mo., cloth, $1 50

PALLETT.—THE MILLER'S, MILLWRIGHT'S, AND ENGINEER'S GUIDE.

By HENRY PALLETT. Illustrated. In one vol. 12mo. . $3 00

PERKINS.—GAS AND VENTILATION.

Practical Treatise on Gas and Ventilation. With Special Relation to Illuminating, Heating, and Cooking by Gas. Including Scientific Helps to Engineer-students and others. With illustrated Diagrams. By E. E. PERKINS. 12mo., cloth . . . $1 25

PERKINS AND STOWE.—A NEW GUIDE TO THE SHEET-IRON AND BOILER PLATE ROLLER:

Containing a Series of Tables showing the Weight of Slabs and Piles to Produce Boiler Plates, and of the Weight of Piles and the Sizes of Bars to Produce Sheet-iron; the Thickness of the Bar Gauge in Decimals; the Weight per foot, and the Thickness on the Bar or Wire Gauge of the fractional parts of an inch; the Weight per sheet, and the Thickness on the Wire Gauge of Sheet-iron of various dimensions to weigh 112 lbs. per bundle; and the conversion of Short Weight into Long Weight, and Long Weight into Short. Estimated and collected by G. H. PERKINS and J. G. STOWE $2 50

PHILLIPS AND DARLINGTON.—RECORDS OF MINING AND METALLURGY:

Or, Facts and Memoranda for the use of the Mine Agent and Smelter. By J. ARTHUR PHILLIPS, Mining Engineer, Graduate of the Imperial School of Mines, France, etc., and JOHN DARLINGTON. Illustrated by numerous engravings. In one vol. 12mo. . $2 00

PRADAL, MALEPEYRE, AND DUSSAUCE.—A COMPLETE TREATISE ON PERFUMERY:

Containing notices of the Raw Material used in the Art, and the Best Formulæ. According to the most approved Methods followed in France, England, and the United States. By M. P. PRADAL, Perfumer-Chemist, and M. F. MALEPEYRE. Translated from the French, with extensive additions, by Prof. H. DUSSAUCE. 8vo. $10

PROTEAUX.—PRACTICAL GUIDE FOR THE MANUFACTURE OF PAPER AND BOARDS.

By A. PROTEAUX, Civil Engineer, and Graduate of the School of Arts and Manufactures, Director of Thiers's Paper Mill, 'Puy-de-Dôme. With additions, by L. S. LE NORMAND. Translated from the French, with Notes, by HORATIO PAINE, A. B., M. D. To which is added a Chapter on the Manufacture of Paper from Wood in the United States, by HENRY T. BROWN, of the "American Artisan." Illustrated by six plates, containing Drawings of Raw Materials, Machinery, Plans of Paper-Mills, etc. etc. 8vo. $5 00

REGNAULT.—ELEMENTS OF CHEMISTRY.

By M. V. REGNAULT. Translated from the French by T. FORREST BENTON, M. D., and edited, with notes, by JAMES C. BOOTH, Melter and Refiner U. S. Mint, and WM. L. FABER, Metallurgist and Mining Engineer. Illustrated by nearly 700 wood engravings. Comprising nearly 1500 pages. In two vols. 8vo., cloth $10 00

REID.—A PRACTICAL TREATISE ON THE MANUFACTURE OF PORTLAND CEMENT:

By HENRY REID, C. E. To which is added a Translation of M. A. Lipowitz's Work, describing a new method adopted in Germany of Manufacturing that Cement. By W. F. REID. Illustrated by plates and wood engravings. 8vo. $7 00

RIFFAULT, VERGNAUD, AND TOUSSAINT.—A PRACTICAL TREATISE ON THE MANUFACTURE OF COLORS FOR PAINTING:

Containing the best Formulæ and the Processes the Newest and in most General Use. By MM. RIFFAULT, VERGNAUD, and TOUSSAINT. Revised and Edited by M. F. MALEPEYRE and Dr. EMIL WINCKLER. Illustrated by Engravings. In one vol. 8vo. (*In preparation.*)

RIFFAULT, VERGNAUD, AND TOUSSAINT.—A PRACTICAL TREATISE ON THE MANUFACTURE OF VARNISHES:

By MM. RIFFAULT, VERGNAUD, and TOUSSAINT. Revised and Edited by M. F. MALEPEYRE and Dr. EMIL WINCKLER. Illustrated. In one vol. 8vo. (*In preparation.*)

SHUNK.—A PRACTICAL TREATISE ON RAILWAY CURVES AND LOCATION, FOR YOUNG ENGINEERS.

By WM. F. SHUNK, Civil Engineer. 12mo., tucks . . $2 00

SMEATON.—BUILDER'S POCKET COMPANION:

Containing the Elements of Building, Surveying, and Architecture; with Practical Rules and Instructions connected with the subject. By A. C. SMEATON, Civil Engineer, etc. In one volume, 12mo. $1 50

SMITH.—THE DYER'S INSTRUCTOR:

Comprising Practical Instructions in the Art of Dyeing Silk, Cotton, Wool, and Worsted, and Woollen Goods: containing nearly 800 Receipts. To which is added a Treatise on the Art of Padding; and the Printing of Silk Warps, Skeins, and Handkerchiefs, and the various Mordants and Colors for the different styles of such work. By DAVID SMITH, Pattern Dyer, 12mo., cloth $3 00

SMITH.—THE PRACTICAL DYER'S GUIDE:

Comprising Practical Instructions in the Dyeing of Shot Cobourgs, Silk Striped Orleans, Colored Orleans from Black Warps, ditto from White Warps, Colored Cobourgs from White Warps, Merinos, Yarns, Woollen Cloths, etc. Containing nearly 300 Receipts, to most of which a Dyed Pattern is annexed. Also, a Treatise on the Art of Padding. By DAVID SMITH. In one vol. 8vo. $25 00

SHAW.—CIVIL ARCHITECTURE:

Being a Complete Theoretical and Practical System of Building, containing the Fundamental Principles of the Art. By EDWARD SHAW, Architect. To which is added a Treatise on Gothic Architecture, &c. By THOMAS W. SILLOWAY and GEORGE M. HARDING, Architects. The whole illustrated by 102 quarto plates finely engraved on copper. Eleventh Edition. 4to. Cloth. $10 00

SLOAN.—AMERICAN HOUSES:

A variety of Original Designs for Rural Buildings. Illustrated by 26 colored Engravings, with Descriptive References. By SAMUEL SLOAN, Architect, author of the "Model Architect," etc. etc. 8vo. $2 50

SCHINZ.—RESEARCHES ON THE ACTION OF THE BLAST-FURNACE.

By CHAS. SCHINZ. Seven plates. 12mo. $4 25

SMITH.—PARKS AND PLEASURE GROUNDS:

Or, Practical Notes on Country Residences, Villas, Public Parks, and Gardens. By CHARLES H. J. SMITH, Landscape Gardener and Garden Architect, etc. etc. 12mo. $2 25

STOKES.—CABINET-MAKER'S AND UPHOLSTERER'S COMPANION:

Comprising the Rudiments and Principles of Cabinet-making and Upholstery, with Familiar Instructions, Illustrated by Examples for attaining a Proficiency in the Art of Drawing, as applicable to Cabinet-work; The Processes of Veneering, Inlaying, and Buhl-work; the Art of Dyeing and Staining Wood, Bone, Tortoise Shell, etc. Directions for Lackering, Japanning, and Varnishing; to make French Polish; to prepare the Best Glues, Cements, and Compositions, and a number of Receipts, particularly for workmen generally. By J. STOKES. In one vol. 12mo. With illustrations $1 25

STRENGTH AND OTHER PROPERTIES OF METALS.

Reports of Experiments on the Strength and other Properties of Metals for Cannon. With a Description of the Machines for Testing Metals, and of the Classification of Cannon in service. By Officers of the Ordnance Department U. S. Army. By authority of the Secretary of War. Illustrated by 25 large steel plates. In 1 vol. quarto $10 00

SULLIVAN.—PROTECTION TO NATIVE INDUSTRY.

By Sir EDWARD SULLIVAN, Baronet. (1870.) 8vo. . $1 50

TABLES SHOWING THE WEIGHT OF ROUND, SQUARE, AND FLAT BAR IRON, STEEL, ETC.

By Measurement. Cloth 63

TAYLOR.—STATISTICS OF COAL:

Including Mineral Bituminous Substances employed in Arts and Manufactures; with their Geographical, Geological, and Commercial Distribution and amount of Production and Consumption on the American Continent. With Incidental Statistics of the Iron Manufacture. By R. C. TAYLOR. Second edition, revised by S. S. HALDEMAN. Illustrated by five Maps and many wood engravings. 8vo., cloth $6 00

TEMPLETON.—THE PRACTICAL EXAMINATOR ON STEAM AND THE STEAM-ENGINE:

With Instructive References relative thereto, for the Use of Engineers, Students, and others. By WM. TEMPLETON, Engineer. 12mo. $1 25

THOMAS.—THE MODERN PRACTICE OF PHOTOGRAPHY.
By R. W. Thomas, F. C. S. 8vo., cloth 75

THOMSON.—FREIGHT CHARGES CALCULATOR.
By Andrew Thomson, Freight Agent $1 25

TURNING: SPECIMENS OF FANCY TURNING EXECUTED ON THE HAND OR FOOT LATHE:
With Geometric, Oval, and Eccentric Chucks, and Elliptical Cutting Frame. By an Amateur. Illustrated by 30 exquisite Photographs. 4to. $3 00

TURNER'S (THE) COMPANION:
Containing Instructions in Concentric, Elliptic, and Eccentric Turning; also various Plates of Chucks, Tools, and Instruments; and Directions for using the Eccentric Cutter, Drill, Vertical Cutter, and Circular Rest; with Patterns and Instructions for working them. A new edition in 1 vol. 12mo. $1 50

URBIN—BRULL.—A PRACTICAL GUIDE FOR PUDDLING IRON AND STEEL.
By Ed. Urbin, Engineer of Arts and Manufactures. A Prize Essay read before the Association of Engineers, Graduate of the School of Mines, of Liege, Belgium, at the Meeting of 1865–6. To which is added a Comparison of the Resisting Properties of Iron and Steel. By A. Brull. Translated from the French by A. A. Fesquet, Chemist and Engineer. In one volume, 8vo. $1 00

VOGDES.—THE ARCHITECT'S AND BUILDER'S POCKET COMPANION AND PRICE BOOK.
By F. W. Vogdes, Architect. Illustrated. Full bound in pocketbook form. $2 00
In book form, 18mo., muslin 1 50

WARN.—THE SHEET METAL WORKER'S INSTRUCTOR, FOR ZINC, SHEET-IRON, COPPER AND TIN PLATE WORKERS, &c.
By Reuben Henry Warn, Practical Tin Plate Worker. Illustrated by 32 plates and 37 wood engravings. 8vo. . . $3 00

WATSON.—A MANUAL OF THE HAND-LATHE.
By Egbert P. Watson, Late of the "Scientific American," Author of "Modern Practice of American Machinists and Engineers," In one volume, 12mo. $1 50

WATSON.—THE MODERN PRACTICE OF AMERICAN MACHINISTS AND ENGINEERS:

Including the Construction, Application, and Use of Drills, Lathe Tools, Cutters for Boring Cylinders, and Hollow Work Generally, with the most Economical Speed of the same, the Results verified by Actual Practice at the Lathe, the Vice, and on the Floor. Together with Workshop management, Economy of Manufacture, the Steam-Engine, Boilers, Gears, Belting, etc. etc. By EGBERT P. WATSON, late of the "Scientific American." Illustrated by eighty-six engravings. 12mo. $2 50

WATSON.—THE THEORY AND PRACTICE OF THE ART OF WEAVING BY HAND AND POWER:

With Calculations and Tables for the use of those connected with the Trade. By JOHN WATSON, Manufacturer and Practical Machine Maker. Illustrated by large drawings of the best Power-Looms. 8vo. $10 00

WEATHERLY.—TREATISE ON THE ART OF BOILING SUGAR, CRYSTALLIZING, LOZENGE-MAKING, COMFITS, GUM GOODS,

And other processes for Confectionery, &c. In which are explained, in an easy and familiar manner, the various Methods of Manufacturing every description of Raw and Refined Sugar Goods, as sold by Confectioners and others . . . $2 00

WILL.—TABLES FOR QUALITATIVE CHEMICAL ANALYSIS.

By Prof. HEINRICH WILL, of Giessen, Germany. Seventh edition. Translated by CHARLES F. HIMES, Ph. D., Professor of Natural Science, Dickinson College, Carlisle, Pa. . . $1 25

WILLIAMS.—ON HEAT AND STEAM:

Embracing New Views of Vaporization, Condensation, and Expansion. By CHARLES WYE WILLIAMS, A. I. C. E. Illustrated. 8vo. $3 50

WORSSAM.—ON MECHANICAL SAWS:

From the Transactions of the Society of Engineers, 1867. By S. W. WORSSAM, Jr. Illustrated by 18 large folding plates. 8vo. $5 00

WOHLER.—A HAND-BOOK OF MINERAL ANALYSIS.

By F. WÖHLER. Edited by H. B. NASON, Professor of Chemistry, Rensselaer Institute, Troy, N. Y. With numerous Illustrations. 12mo. $3 00

www.ingramcontent.com/pod-product-compliance
Lightning Source LLC
LaVergne TN
LVHW020119110826
845151LV00001B/212

* 9 7 8 1 4 2 5 5 4 1 7 9 8 *